Julie Tominaga MD
530-756-4327

D0437586

The
Young
Athlete

The Young Athlete

A SPORTS DOCTOR'S COMPLETE GUIDE FOR PARENTS

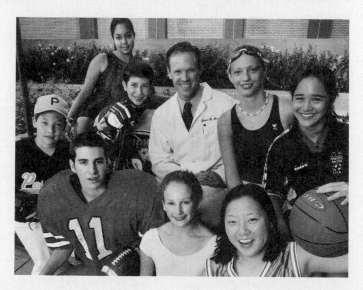

Jordan D. Metzl, M.D., and Carol Shookhoff

Little, Brown and Company

Boston · New York · London

Copyright © 2002 by Jordan D. Metzl, M.D., and Carol Suen Shookhoff

All rights reserved. No part of this book may be reproduced in any form or by any electronic or mechanical means, including information storage and retrieval systems, without permission in writing from the publisher, except by a reviewer who may quote brief passages in a review.

First Edition

This book is not intended as a substitute for the medical advice of physicians. The reader should regularly consult a physician in all matters relating to his or her child's health, and particularly with respect to any symptoms that may require diagnosis or medical attention.

Library of Congress Cataloging-in-Publication Data
Metzl, Jordan D.
The young athlete : a sports doctor's complete guide for parents / by Jordan D. Metzl and Carol Shookhoff. — 1st ed.
p. cm.
Includes bibliographical references and index.
ISBN 0-316-60756-8
1. Sports for children.   2. Sports injuries in children — Prevention.
3. Sports for children — Safety measures.   4. Pediatric sports medicine.
I. Shookhoff, Carol.   II. Title.
GV709.2 .M47 2002
613.7'042 — dc21   2001050562

10 9 8 7 6 5 4 3 2 1

Drawings by Mona Mark

Designed by Chris Welch

Q-FF

Printed in the United States of America

Title page photograph: Scott LaFever (baseball player); Danielle Bolling (gymnast); Gregory Schwedock (hockey player); Alex Goldberger (football player); Jessica Seigel (ballet dancer); Caitlin Olmstead (swimmer); Jenny Werts (basketball player); Alexandra Shookhoff (soccer player)

This book is dedicated to the millions of parents who are working to keep sports healthy, fun, and safe for their children. May it aid you in your efforts.

With love and thanks for their tireless support: Drs. Kurt, Marilyn, Jonathan, Jamie, and soon-to-be-doctor Joshua Metzl, and David and Alexandra Shookhoff.

In 1934 I coined my own definition for success, which I tried to personally attain and get all my students to attain. It is "peace of mind," which is a direct result of self-satisfaction in knowing you did your best to become the best of which you are capable.

— *John Wooden, UCLA basketball coach, 1948–75*

Contents

x   Contents

Preface

The past fifteen years have seen a youth sports explosion in the United States. Currently, more than 30 million children and teens under the age of eighteen participate in some form of organized sports, and the number keeps rising. Sports are also becoming more competitive. We are seeing kids as young as seven and eight on "travel" and "select" teams, playing high-level, competitive sports year-round. For better or worse, the old days of just tossing a ball around in the backyard are gone.

For parents, this phenomenon has created an array of bewildering new questions. Parents and kids know that sports are supposed to be fun, build leadership and social skills, and provide many health benefits. But is there such a thing as too much? How can parents recognize when sports are potentially injurious, and how can they keep participation safe and healthy? How can they ensure that their kids are receiving proper training and coaching and are developing the kinds of positive values that sports are supposed to instill? How can they make certain that sports remain enjoyable, rewarding, and safe; contribute to the overall development of their child; and in general represent "value added" in the life of their child?

I have written this book to help provide parents with answers to these questions.

The Young Athlete: A Sports Doctor's Complete Guide for Parents gives the most current information about safe sports participation for kids. The information is applicable to the young athlete at all levels, from the child just starting peewee sports to the advanced-level high school player contemplating a college career. The book covers both parenting and medical issues. There is also a chapter on development that addresses specific health concerns for male and female athletes.

✳

In many ways, this book is the story of my life.

People often ask me, "How did you become a sports medicine doctor?" My desire to be a doctor dates back as far as I can remember. Healing others was a way of life in my family. My pediatrician father has always been a role model for me. When I was little, I would visit his office and see how he took care of kids and their families. But when it came time for my own blood tests and immunizations, he literally had to chase me, screaming at the top of my lungs, down the hall. Nonetheless, I found the smell of his office familiar and comforting. My mother is a psychologist who treats teens and their families, helping them explore the issues behind their behavior patterns. Walking down the street in Kansas City, I often run into people who say, "Your mom [or your dad] is my doctor. She [or he] is great."

Another prominent force in our family was sports. My parents recount how before I was born, they prepared my one-and-a-half-year-old brother Jonathan to share the limelight with a younger sibling. But when they brought me home, Jonathan took one look at me, waved, and then tried to sit on my head. Two years after I was born, a third son, Jamie, rounded out the first wave of Metzl sons.

With three boys born within four years of each other, testosterone abounded in the Metzl household. Each boy wanted to play well, and in particular, better than his brothers. We competed in everything, from who could draw the best picture to who could hit the most free throws. I remember waking up at seven o'clock on Sundays to play cutthroat Wiffle ball in the backyard with my brothers. These games were for glory. Chasing a long fly ball, I once crashed into the woodpile and broke a toe. I remember heated one-on-one basketball games almost every summer evening, played under a halogen light with crickets chirping in the background. Team sports were also important, particularly Little League baseball. Making a good play meant you could walk tall around the house.

My parents didn't want to raise just "dumb jocks." They took us to the ballet, opera, and theater; family discussions were more often about politics or books than sports. We all played musical instruments, though I sometimes used my flute as a baseball bat for Nerf-baseball games in my bedroom.

When I was a teenager, my parents decided to have another child. I regarded the little newcomer, Josh, as my sports project. I spent hours teaching him to throw, hit a fastball, shoot a basketball. Josh has just graduated from college, and when we run marathons together he laughs as he speeds past me.

As I grew older, sports continued to shape my life. In college, I played varsity soccer; in medical school, I did triathlons; and in residency, I started running marathons. I needed time on the field as much as in the classroom. Sports and exercise gave me a sense of community with my teammates and the other athletes on campus.

Sports also helped me burn off extra energy so I could study better at night. Many people seem to need to burn off energy in order to concentrate. Maybe that's why athletes tend to do better academically during their sports season. The medical profession can't explain exactly why this is, but it's a recognized phenomenon, and I know personally that physical activity makes a huge difference to my mental focus.

As my medical training progressed, I knew I had to find a way to combine my two passions, athletics and medicine. Many people, especially in the highly academic Boston medical community, scoffed at the idea of sports medicine; many considered it lowbrow. But I believed that sports and medicine complement each other. The patients I most enjoyed taking care of were the athletic kids. They came to the Boston clinic where I did my residency saying, "I want to get back to sports as soon as I can. It's important for me." I completely understood what they were saying. Plus I'd had most of their injuries myself, so I knew exactly how they felt.

After Boston, I got a sports medicine fellowship at Vanderbilt University in Nashville. Here was real sports medicine, behind the scenes of college sports. Before, I had always been on the field as an athlete, working hard to play my best and help my team win. Now I was a doctor, there to make sure that the safest decisions were made for kids playing on all of the sports teams. I had to tell the soccer coach that a player with a concussion could not return to the game, even though the player was eager and willing and so was the coach. The responsibility was sobering. Next I went to Harvard for a second year of sports medicine training, with a focus on adolescents. While there, I interned with the Boston Ballet and learned firsthand about the physical demands of dance, and also about dancers' special medical needs, which are different from those of the average athlete.

Finally, at age thirty-two, when most of my friends had mortgage payments and were on their second or third jobs, I finished my medical training and got my first "grownup" job. I joined the sports medicine division at one of the most reputable orthopedic institutions in the world, the Hospital for Special Surgery (HSS) in New York City. (Yet another relocation!) Staying up all those nights during residency was really worth the effort; I could finally start my own practice.

I have been so happy at HSS, sharing information and helping my patients get back to activity. When a senior football player broke his thumb right before the last game of the season, I came in over the weekend to make him a special cast so that he could finish out his high school career. (He's now a college senior and still writes me with updates about his college football career.) Recently, HSS opened its Sports Medicine Institute for Young Athletes, an integrated sports medicine center that treats, researches, and, we hope, will one day prevent sports injuries in children and teens. As the medical director, I am helping to develop educational programs for coaches and parents to make sports safer for kids.

When a young pitcher, soccer player, or figure skater comes to see me, I understand what sports mean to that young athlete, and to the parents as well. Although a sports injury might not seem like such a big deal in the grand scheme of life, I know that sports help these young people define who they are, and that sports contribute to their physical and emotional development. Only one or two of these athletes will go on to become professionals, but when they are injured, they just want to get back to their sport and their team as soon as they can. Getting them back is important to me because it's important to them.

In academic circles, sports medicine is no longer "lowbrow," but a valid career path with fellowship programs. Pediatric residents come through my office seeking advice and instruction. I feel I'm inspiring them to take better care of their patients, and it's very gratifying to pass my education on to other, younger physicians. I also write, lecture, and teach about sports medicine to parents, coaches, and physicians.

With the growth of my career, I am constantly brought back to the days of playing basketball under the halogen light in our Kansas City backyard. Every Little League player reminds me of dusty afternoons on the baseball diamond, my parents in the stands, me trying to prove my mettle, the nervous energy of each at bat, the joy of making a good play, like the diving catch I made in center field when I was ten. I still remember the flight of the ball, and my utter delight when I stood up holding it in my hand. Each teenage soccer player reminds me of my victories and defeats in high school sports. I remember losing in the district soccer game as a high school senior and feeling as if the whole world were collapsing. Although I now have a more mature perspective (I hope), the challenges of high school sports helped me grow. In the process of combining physical work and mental toughness to push myself to the limit and then try to go beyond, I learned, and still learn, much about myself.

I still play, and still try athletic feats that push me to, and sometimes beyond, my limits. As in the early days, my three brothers are not only my best friends, but also my athletic compatriots. This year, Jamie convinced me to do an Ironman triathlon: a 2.4-mile swim, followed by a 112-mile bicycle ride, and then a marathon of 26.2 miles. It was the ultimate test of my physical and mental self. After ten hours of muttered curses, wondering "Why am I doing this?," I didn't want to move. It was the hardest thing I had ever done. But I knew that finishing was important. For the next two and a half hours, I willed myself to the finish line. When I crossed it, at twelve and a half hours, I was exhilarated because I had defined a new boundary for myself. (Jamie beat me by eleven minutes, so we'll probably do another Ironman sometime not too far off.)

The lessons from sports apply to life in general. Pushing toward a goal, striving for extra courage and strength, is what has allowed me to succeed, both as a person and as a physician.

My doctor parents encouraged all four Metzl sons to be the best athletes and best people they could be. In sports, as in life, they have always been there for us. Despite their busy schedules, they were almost always in the stands for me and each of my brothers. The number of games they sat though is unbelievable.

Looking back, I begin to see how my life as a young athlete and as a member of my family led me to become a sports medicine doctor. This book combines where I have been with where I am now. I hope that you, the parents of young athletes, find its information useful as you encourage your children to be the best that they can be, both on and off the field.

Jordan D. Metzl, M.D.
Medical Director, The Sports Medicine
Institute for Young Athletes
Hospital for Special Surgery
New York, New York

Acknowledgments

The Young Athlete came into being when Carol Shookhoff visited my office two years ago with her injured soccer-playing daughter, Alexandra. She became my associate writer, and her remarkable insights have been invaluable in shaping the book.

The following people were tremendously helpful in the development of our manuscript: Steve Bluth, Melissa Grossfeld, R.D., Shari Bilt, R.D., David Shookhoff, Denise Adorante, Marilyn Lunnetta, Kay Hanson, Ted Bracken, Nancy Hargrave Meislahn, Chris Lanser, Jon Reider, Ray Selvadurai, Lizanne Coyne, Jan Ryan, Laura Clark, Russell Warren, M.D., Robert Marx, M.D., Lyle Micheli, M.D., Paul Stricker, M.D., Kurt Spindler, M.D., and T. J. and Marilyn Suen.

We would also like to thank the following:

Astrid Baumgardner, Don Betterton, Kerry Townsend Bouchier, Jennie Bracken, Maggie Bradley, Monique Breindel, Lisa Callahan, M.D., Geoffrey Chepiga, Eileen Coogan, R.N., Don Farmer, Harry Feder, Cody Foss, ATC, Gale Frederick, Charlie Galbraith, David Hooks, Katrina Jackiewicz, Esq., Chris Kennedy, Larry Lawrence, RuthAnn and Dennis Lobo, Ralph Lopez, M.D., Herb Mack, Andrea Marks, M.D., Tonia Maschi, ATC, Shelly Mayer,

John McCarthy, Jonathan Oberman, Daniel Overmeyer, Cynthia Pegler, M.D., Philip Pizzo, M.D., Dan Roock, Karen Rosewater, M.D., Leo Rutman, Rosemarie Sachetti, Richard Saphir, M.D., Marci Schneider, M.D., Alexandra Shookhoff, Joseph R. Smith, Lee Smith, Chris Sowlakis, ATC, Billy Stampur, Ron Stratten, Ted Suen, Sue Wasiolek, CeCe Waters, Ellen Werts, and Harvey Yancey.

The
Young
Athlete

Chapter 1

The Benefits of Youth Sports

MENS SANA IN CORPORE SANO (A SOUND MIND IN A SOUND BODY)

Sports are for fun, but they also offer benefits and lessons that carry over into all aspects of life.

When kids are asked why they play sports, here's what they say:

- To have fun
- To improve their skills
- To learn new skills
- To be with their friends
- To make new friends
- To succeed or win
- To become physically fit

Kids usually get the benefits they seek from sports and more. Kids need attention and respect (in that order), but they have few ways to get them. What is unique about sports is that they offer kids an arena where they can earn attention and respect by exerting their natural abilities. Kids are good at sports because sports are essentially about speed, strength, coordination, vision, creativity, and

3

responsiveness — the necessary physical attributes are the attributes of youth.

Given that athletics involves all aspects of the human being, it is not surprising that participants benefit in all of the areas they mention. According to researchers at the Institute for the Study of Youth Sports at Michigan State University, kids who participate in organized sports do better in school, have better interpersonal skills, are more team oriented, and are generally healthier.

Participation in sports provides opportunities for leadership and socialization, as well as the development of skills for handling success and failure.

Moreover, when playing games, children learn how rules work. They see how groups need rules to keep order, that the individual must accept the rules for the good of the group, that rules entail a consideration of the rights of others. They also learn about competition, but within a restricted and safe system where the consequences of losing are minimized.

Benefits for girls have been of particular interest to researchers. The President's Council on Physical Fitness and Sports reports many developmental benefits of participating in youth sports for girls, including increased self-esteem and self-confidence, healthier body image, significant experiences of competency and success, as well as reduced risk of chronic disease. Furthermore, female athletes "do better academically and have lower school dropout rates than their nonathletic counterparts."

The Women's Sports Foundation lists many ways that sports specifically benefit female athletes. These include their being less likely to become pregnant as teenagers, less likely to begin smoking, more likely to quit smoking, more likely to do well in science, and more likely to graduate from high school and college than female nonathletes. Female athletes also take greater pride in their physical and social selves than their sedentary peers; they are more active physically as they age; they suffer less depression. There is also some evidence that recreational physical activity decreases a woman's chances of developing breast cancer and helps prevent osteoporosis.

I am convinced that sports offer a unique arena in which children can successfully exert their talents. The arena is unique for two reasons. First, sports engage the child as a complete human being: all facets — not just physical, but also social, cognitive, and psychological — are engaged harmoniously in striving toward peak fulfillment. Second, sports involve youths working in an ongoing community composed of their peers as well as their peers' families. Sports, that is, offer children an exhilarating, satisfying, rewarding way to participate in a larger world not generally accessible to nonathletes.

Physical Benefits

- **Fitness.** Kids who play sports develop general physical fitness in a way that's fun, and they establish lifelong habits for good health. This is particularly important at a time when obesity in the United States has reached epidemic proportions: the incidence of obesity has increased by more than 50 percent among America's children and teens since 1976 and continues to grow at a staggering rate!
- **Stress relief.** Sports allow kids to clear their minds of academic and social pressures, to literally run off the tension that's accumulated in their muscles. In the words of one patient, "If you play really hard, you feel better because playing takes your mind off things that bother you, and afterwards you can concentrate better." Most doctors recognize the positive mental effect of physical exertion, even though we're not sure exactly why this is so. I know that my ability to study in college and medical school was greatly enhanced when I ran during the day, and I'm not the only athlete to find this true. Many athletes get better grades in-season (theories posit the discipline and the need to manage

time, along with an increased ability to concentrate). During exams, Duke University opens its gyms twenty-four hours a day to provide stress relief for its students.

- **Mastery.** Sports give kids a satisfying, enjoyable way to develop their own talents: through personal effort they get good at something they're interested in. Doing something well makes them feel good about themselves, but equally important, it teaches them about the process of how to improve and work more effectively. Learning a skill — to dribble left-handed, say, or to execute an effective second serve — entails a recognition that practice is essential and that improvement is incremental. The process of repetition teaches the athlete how to master a move and also how to experiment with different approaches to improve a skill. The feedback in sports is usually immediate and visible — does the ball go into the basket? — so that the athlete can change or repeat what she's doing and figure out how to get better. Not only that, the whole process of seeing practice lead to improvement gives kids a feeling of control, a feeling all too rare in their lives.

- **Healthy habits.** Because sports increase an awareness of one's body and how it responds to different stimuli and circumstances, sports help prevent drug and alcohol abuse. Most athletes value what their bodies can do and want to maintain those abilities. Being an athlete also gives kids an acceptable reason for telling their friends no to drugs, booze, and other high-risk, unhealthy behaviors. (Of course, not all athletes avoid drugs and alcohol.)

Personal Benefits

- **Valuing preparation.** Sports help kids learn to distinguish between effort and ability. Sports increase self-discipline and the awareness of the value of preparation because kids can see the difference in their performance.

Competitive athletes learn the importance of effort, being prepared (mentally and physically), and enlightened risk-taking. They see that raw physical talent is not always sufficient to win the game, but that preparation is essential. This includes mental preparation (staying focused) and physical fitness as well as practicing the plays with their teammates in team sports. They learn to evaluate risk versus reward. Another invaluable lesson is discovering that mistakes are part of learning; they signal that a particular approach is unsuccessful and you must try another. Kids also learn to deal productively with criticism as part of improvement and preparation.

• **Resilience.** Sports provide an unparalleled model for dealing with disappointment and misfortune. Young athletes learn to handle adversity, whether it's picking themselves up after losing a big game or not getting as many minutes as they wanted. They find ways to deal with losing and go on, because there's another big game next week or next year. They figure out what to do to get what they want for themselves. They put in extra time on fitness or work on specific weaknesses in their game (long-ball trapping, hitting to the opposite field, looking the ball into their hands).

Athletes also learn to deal with the physical and psychological effects of injury. I broke my jaw playing soccer and missed most of the season my junior year in high school. I went through the classic stages of grief, from "This can't be true" to ultimate acceptance. Two months of sitting out, waiting to heal, and dealing with physical and emotional pain was devastating. There were times early on when I sat in my bed whimpering from pain. But as time went on and my jaw began to heal, I somehow began to realize what almost all athletes in pain realize: the only person who is going to help you is yourself. You find the limits of what you can ask of yourself and know that you will deliver. This learning to get the best out of yourself carries over into all aspects of life. People can find their internal drive through training and hard work, but adversity really brings it out. In my case, I came back with stronger resolve. In my senior year I became an all-district soccer player and was propelled toward a college soccer career.

- **Attitude control.** Older teens learn that a confident attitude improves their performance, and that they have some control over their attitude. They learn to disregard comparative stats in preparing for an opponent and instead to adopt "attitude enhancers" such as visualization exercises, team or individual rituals, singing specific songs together, or having dinner as a team the night before the game. Some might call these superstitions, others, self-fulfilling prophecies, but they work.

- **Leadership opportunities.** Team sports offer kids a rare opportunity to serve as leaders. Kids can be in a position to assess the strengths and weaknesses of their various teammates and help to exploit their strengths and compensate for their weaknesses. They can minimize conflicts among players. They can reinforce values — such as fair play, teamsmanship, hard work, mental preparation — by speaking up when appropriate and setting a good example. They can also take the initiative in arranging for team dress on game days (football players wear their jerseys to class, female basketball players wear their warm-up pants), organizing team dinners or team movie nights, and inviting teachers and administrators to their games.

- **Identity and balance.** Being part of a group is inordinately important to kids, and sports make kids feel like they belong, whether it's to the group of athletes in general or their team in particular. Sports also contribute to a teenager's sense of a stable identity with particular values. "I'm a football player" is a very different statement than "I play football." People are complicated, however; no individual is just one thing. It's better to encourage children — and adults — not to assume a single identity to the exclusion of all else.

- **Time management.** Young athletes learn to manage their time productively. They know they have to get their homework done, so they learn not to waste time (some of them even quit watching television and hanging out at the mall). They plan ahead, so that big school projects don't catch them by surprise. They even figure out they have to eat well and get a good night's sleep. Countless athletes, in school and the workplace, say that being an athlete taught them discipline that is invaluable in their lives on and off the field.

- **Long-term thinking.** Athletes learn the fundamental lesson of sacrificing immediate gratification for long-term gain. This is the basis for personal success as well as for civilization in general, and no lesson can be more valuable.

Social Benefits

Sports are a social activity. Team sports are obviously done with other people, but even individual sports are often done as a team (tennis, golf, track). All sports, however, are intended to be performed in front of others, and the social ramifications are many. Here are some of them.

- **Relationships with other kids.** Athletes develop relationships with their teammates. For boys, sports are a primary, and unfortunately sometimes the sole, way of socializing with others. In many schools and communities, nonathletic males find it difficult to develop a social network at all. For girls, who according to the feminist theorist Carol Gilligan tend to define themselves through their relationships rather than their achievements, sports offer yet another way to make friends and create an alternate peer group. According to Mike Nerney, a consultant in substance abuse prevention and education, multiple peer groups are always a good idea for teens, who have an intense need for inclusion and belonging, but who can also be volatile, cruel to each other, and foment destructive behavior as a group. Having a refuge when relations go wrong with one group can alleviate a great deal of stress and offer an alternative for kids who feel uncomfortable or frightened by peers who engage in high-risk activities.

- **Teamwork.** On a team, kids learn about cooperation, camaraderie, give-and-take. They learn that while their natural position might be wide receiver, the team needs a cornerback, so they sacrifice their personal desires and play defense. They learn that you don't have to like someone in order to work together toward a common goal. They also discover that you can work for people you don't respect and still be productive, improve your skills, and have fun. A team is a natural environment in which to learn responsibility to others: you can't stay out carousing the night before a game; sometimes you need to pass up a party in order to show up and play well.

  Kids learn these lessons from their teammates and, most important, a coach who encourages the good of the team over the needs of an individual player. This attitude is sometimes rare in today's sports climate, where what's glorified is to "be the man." I think the earlier the message is instilled about the good of the larger whole, the better for kids in the long run.

- **Diversity.** Organized sports sponsored by clubs or youth leagues not affiliated with schools offer players an opportunity to meet a variety of kids from different backgrounds. Students from public, private, and parochial schools come together in a common enterprise, crossing socioeconomic and ethnic lines, so that over time all players broaden their sense of how other people live. The genuinely multicultural environment is of tremendous importance in our polarized society. Kids play on the same team, wear the same uniform, share the same objectives and experiences. Sports are a great equalizer: rich or poor, black, brown, or white, are irrelevant. What counts is talent and heart.

- **Relationships with adults.** When coaches, parents, and kids see each other at practice and games week after week, year after year, the adults learn to admire and praise the kids' prowess and progress, even when kids are as young as third graders. This kind of attention helps youngsters learn to balance their own evaluation of their improving skills with the appraisal of others who are not blood relatives; they also begin the lifelong process of figuring out whom to listen to when they hear conflicting advice or assessments. In addition, for young athletes of all ages, attention from interested adults is not only flattering but also helps them overcome shyness and develop poise when talking to relative strangers in social situations. The ability to feel comfortable in a variety of social circumstances will be progressively more valuable in a world of multiple cultures and decreasing numbers of supportive communities.

Sports give kids an opportunity to spend ongoing periods of time with an adult in a shared endeavor. Indeed, kids may spend more time with their coach than with any other adult in their lives, especially if they're on a school team or a club team that practices two or more times a week. Ideally this coach cares about them as whole beings rather than particular talents who can run for touchdowns or block opponents' shots. To thrive, kids need to be with adults who want them to do well in a variety of endeavors, who notice their improvements and hard work, who manifest sound values, and who don't pay attention to them solely because of their contributions to the win column.

The coach–player relationship can be very strong, and even parentlike. Coaches of young athletes take on a tremendous responsibility to set a good example and treat their players respectfully. Thankfully, most coaches take this responsibility very seriously.

Sometimes, the coach–player relationship can even be lifesaving. A female coach of a varsity boys' team reported that one of her players came to her saying, "I need to talk to you. I found blood in my urine."

"Let me ask you something," the coach replied. "Have you been having unprotected sex?"

"No, of course not. I can't believe you asked me that," he said.

"Well, I need to know what direction to take you in. No matter what happened, you need to see a doctor."

The coach recalled, "This boy was very good looking and very popular. I knew what was going on. The doctor found he had picked up a venereal disease which could have made him infertile. The boy called me from the doctor's office to say thank you."

• **Participating in a community.** Sports foster a sense of community: they give both participants and spectators the experience of belonging to something larger than themselves, the need for which seems to be hard-wired into the human brain. This is why kids love playing for their schools, why high school football games in small cities can draw tens of thousands of spectators week after week, and why adults identify with their college teams years after they have graduated. Playing for an institution or a community gives kids a chance to feel that they are making a genuine contribution to a larger group.

Highs and Lows

Sports can actually change the physiology of athletes and fans. Physical exertion can raise the level of pheronemes and endorphins, brain chemicals that cause exhilaration. Exercise can also elevate the serum testosterone level, which makes the heart beat faster. Spectators can feel depressed when their team loses and elated when their team wins. They, too, undergo physiological changes when watching their team: fans of the winning team experience an increase in testosterone, whereas supporters of the losers undergo a decrease in testosterone.

When playing for school or club teams, young athletes are afforded the opportunity to see how grownups and children treat one another and how this treatment has long-term consequences. They can see which adults care about kids, are willing to do their fair share and more, and take a stand for what they believe in. They see which parents are cooperative — pitching in to help with snacks, driving their kids' teammates to games, serving as team treasurer, volunteering to line the fields on cold, rainy mornings. They hear parents screaming at the officials and recognize which ones know the rules and which don't. They see who supports their own children and others, who bullies their children or the officials. They see parents who teach their children to assume they are always right, are better than the other players, and that someone else, anyone else, is always at fault if things go wrong. They also see how the kids in these families emulate or reject their parents' behavior. They think about how they will treat their own children and how they will behave with their friends as members of groups.

One hockey father says, "Part of the benefit of sports is that children observe its complex social dynamic among coaches, parents, players, and officials. There's a wide range of ethics, such as the attitude toward authority. Do you try to abide by the spirit of the rules, get away with what you can, accept what an official says, or do you argue and yell at him, or complain about it? Another major element they encounter is the difference between teammates who are good at communicating and sharing versus those who are out to get what they can for themselves. This is a dichotomy adults face throughout life. Kids involved in sports have to consciously or subconsciously figure out where they fit into those various spectrums."

Participating for years on the same team not only improves the play, because the players learn each other's strengths and weaknesses and where they'll be on the field or court, but it gives kids a wider view of the world and the people in it.

Similarities of Sports and the Arts

Are the benefits of sports unique? Many have noted that the arts produce many of the same benefits as sports, for both participant and spectator.

Sports entail all elements of human life — physical, emotional, cognitive, social — but in a simplified, orderly form. Sports boil life down to competition governed by agreed-upon rules. The opponents are known, the goals clear and quantifiable. Athletes practice the skills necessary to excel and gain a sense of control and mastery. Sports are a public performance, which fosters a sense of community among people — participants as well as spectators — who would otherwise be strangers. At their best, they produce a sense of exhilaration.

The arts are the other significant leisure activity that distills life down to simpler forms. The arts simplify life by selecting and arranging certain elements to create a unified, expressive whole. They too are intended for an audience. The performing arts, dance in particular, have much in common with sports: they take place outside of everyday life, the activities are physical and demand practice, and performance can produce exhilaration and a sense of community.

What makes sports different from the arts is that they demand a spontaneous response to surprise. A dance is choreographed; the dancers know what they are to do at every moment. A game has set plays, but the athletes must respond to what their opponents do, or to the unexpected bounce of the ball. The denouement of the game is uncertain, often until its final seconds. This combination of total human exertion with an environment that balances control, spontaneity, and uncertainty leads to the unique excitement and satisfaction of sports, for both athletes and spectators.

✳

As with most spheres of human endeavor, the benefits of sports can easily turn into deficits. Moderation is, as the Greeks pointed out, the key to wisdom. Many in the athletic community worry that youth sports have become too serious, and that the win-at-all-costs mentality has become the reality today. Youth sports shouldn't be an obsession that excludes other areas of life (academics, the arts, community service, family life, religious training). Sports should be just one arena of many in which kids have a chance to express themselves and have fun.

When winning is overvalued, the idea of sportsmanship and fair play disappears, as does concern for the whole child. When only a kid's athletic talent is important, her character development, her academic performance and needs, her long-term physical health, the development of her skills at other positions on a team are neglected. The pressure to be a winner may push some young athletes toward unsafe performance-enhancing drugs or body-building supplements. Furthermore, when winning is the prime value, the public nature of sports can turn sour. An athlete who is not playing well or makes a mistake may feel humiliation and shame because she knows everyone is watching.

Being a member of a team can become destructive if the players turn arrogant and fall into an us–them mentality, seeing opponents as the enemy and treating their nonathletic peers as inferior or contemptible. Furthermore, if a teenager overidentifies as an athlete, he will be ignoring other interests at a time when he should be broadening rather than narrowing his horizons.

College and professional sports have become corrupted by the win-at-all-costs mentality, and this corruption is intensified by big-money contracts for winning players, coaches, and organizations. Loyalty, camaraderie, sportsmanship, the joy of mastering skills — these values all too often disappear when "winning is the only thing." If they remain uninfected by the toxins of winning at all costs and instead focus on effort and fair play, youth sports can be beautiful, exciting, and fun. They can provide kids with an extraordinary opportunity to express their talents and their character, to run around screaming and laughing with joy.

The job of parents and coaches of young athletes is to maximize the benefits and minimize the deficits of youth sports by keeping a long-term perspective and helping kids do the same.

The Box Score

- The benefits of youth sports are physical, personal, and social.
- The deficits of youth sports are physical, personal, and social.
- Adults make the difference, for good or ill.
- Moderation and balance in all things.

Chapter 2

Life on the Sidelines

BEING A GOOD SPORTS PARENT

*Being a good sports parent means supporting your child's needs,
setting a good example, and being respectful to the people who make
sports possible: the coaches, officials, other parents, and the kids.*

f you're involved in youth sports, then you already know the horror
stories:

- The father who berates a teenage ref, "You idiot! You just *think*
  you're a man because you have a whistle in your mouth, but you
  don't even know the rules!"
- The father who yanks his daughter out of a tournament game,
  then swings at the coach, screaming, "You're not giving Lisa
  enough playing time but you keep your own kid in the whole
  game!" while Lisa weeps with embarrassment.
- The mother who screams at her child that she isn't kicking or tack-
  ling hard enough, isn't shooting often enough. The girl freezes up
  and plays well only when her mother doesn't attend the game.
- The father who tells the coach to yell at his child for "losing" the
  game, because "it builds character."
- The father (who's not the coach) who walks out to the pitching
  mound and tells his ten-year-old son, loudly enough for all the

17

players and parents to hear, "I'm not going to let you pitch any-more. You've embarrassed yourself enough today."

Then there are the extreme cases: fathers, and mothers too, who engage in criminal assault, such as the father who menaced a teenage ref with a knife, or the father who killed his son's youth hockey coach when they got in a fight over the coach's encouraging the players to be overly physical.

Athletics can also, however, bring out the best in parents. There are shining-moments stories aplenty:

- The parent-coach of an eight-year-olds' soccer team who risks losing a game (and incurring parental wrath) by telling the ref the opposing team had scored a goal the ref hadn't seen.
- The mother who tells the coach it's okay to bench her child because he didn't attend a mandatory practice.
- The mother who cheers all good plays, whether made by her own child, a teammate, or someone from the opposing team.
- The father who thanks an umpire for doing a good job.
- The parents who volunteer to do whatever the team or league needs to have done: set up the fields, manage the scheduling of officials, design and order uniforms, organize a fund-raising bake sale, sign up parents to bring snacks for the players, distribute driving directions.

Get a Handle on Your Own Issues

Being a good parent on the sidelines is complicated. While a few rules are absolute — courtesy, respect for others, good sportsman-ship — other guidelines depend on particular circumstances, such as the age and talent of the child, what the child wants, what the parent wants, and the fit between the desires and expectations of parent and child.

When a child begins to play organized sports (often by age five), the parent can sometimes find himself reliving his own youthful fantasies; he envisions Johnny sinking a basket from half-court at the buzzer to win the game, just like he did (or worse, didn't) in high school. The parent of a novice athlete is also customarily afflicted by a host of unexpected and difficult emotions, ranging from feeling judged by outsiders to wanting the child to have fun and learn, but also wanting the child to excel.

Sports Start Early

Recreational leagues have different ages for joining up.

- AYSO (American Youth Soccer Organization) soccer begins at age 5.
- T-ball begins at 4 or 5.
- Pop Warner football starts at 7 or 8.
- Peewee ice hockey leagues start at 7 or 8.

Several studies have shown that injury rates to athletes under age 12 (that is, before puberty) are quite low. Most kids' sports are safe.

It is very difficult to resist the impulse to compare our children to others. When a child enters a group situation such as school or organized sports, parents are often confronted with their first experience of seeing a large number of the same children repeatedly. The human brain learns by comparing and contrasting. On the one hand, it is comforting to see other children being just as annoying (whining, defiant, bossy, impudent) as ours. On the other hand, it's devastating to see other children being "better" than our own — more articulate, creative, knowledgeable, polite, and so on. The pressure on parents is enormous. They want their children to do well, and they know they are being judged by the behavior and abilities of their children, whether this is fair or not. In addition, any parent who wants to can easily find areas where they can call themselves deficient. I see a lot of parents berating themselves — for "saying the wrong thing" to their child or "not being supportive enough." I remind them: You don't have to be perfect. You just have to be right most of the time (meaning over 50 percent and trying for higher), set a good example, and make sure your kids know you're on their side.

This need to compare is real and has consequences. The pressures aroused by feelings of competition and parental inadequacy intensify when a child begins to play organized sports. Sports are defined by certain measurable expectations and criteria about performance, so children get judged for their "talent" — even though at age five or six, sheer size and aggressiveness usually make more difference than coordination and technical ability. Sports often begin at the same time the child enters school, so the pressures sometimes feel exponential.

On top of all this, the sports environment is unpredictable and very public (remember, they're called *"spectator* sports"). You find you have almost no control over what your children will be subjected to. Sports can provide new language other kids can use to torment poor Janie ("*She* can't hit the ball"). Meanwhile, you have to stand supportively on the sidelines, alongside other viewing parents and children, unable to protect Janie from possible insult and humiliation. And if the child is very young, you may have had little experience and time to reflect on your own feelings and how best to help your child in these new circumstances of being appraised by friends and total strangers for her ability to win or at least score.

The Competition Factor

In life, there are many ways to win. A child can grow up to become an engineer, a writer, a doctor. Most parents would be very pleased by any one of these outcomes. But in sports, when one side wins, the other side loses. Indeed, winning is defined as beating the opposition. All too often, a broader idea of success — being the best that you can be, fulfilling your potential, improving your skills, doing something you love, building character and perseverance — is completely forgotten.

Parents want their children to have fun and learn new skills. On the other hand, they also want their children to be outstanding at whatever they pursue (that is, to be better than their peers) and to learn to compete aggressively so as to better navigate their way in the wider world. They want them to win — in sports and in life. The more competitive the parents, the more they want that win — for themselves as well as for their child.

Athletic competition seems to be particularly acute for men, who tend to define themselves through external achievement. Sports, which some see as a healthy alternative to battle, provide an arena in which to achieve visible, measurable, and lauded success. Sports also provide an opportunity for humiliation and embarrassment. I hear too many stories of grownups recalling the searing pain of losing a game as a child and being blamed in public, or private, by their parents. Of grownups who stopped playing a sport they loved because they felt too much pressure to excel and win.

One father I know, I'll call him Jake, normally the nicest guy in the world, sometimes transforms into a terror at basketball games when his daughter is playing. Jake's father was a professional player. Jake played as a kid, and his father criticized him mercilessly and incessantly until Jake finally had the good sense to quit. Now Jake wants to support his daughter's athletic efforts but also wants her to be "the best." He harasses refs with his bitter, barking criticism and has trained his daughter to blame her teammates for any mistakes she makes on the court. Unwittingly he has set up the same dynamic with his daughter that his father did with him: making basketball unpleasant by hewing to unrealistic judgments. He needs to step back and gain a wider perspective on how his attitude is warping his daughter's self-esteem and her relations with other people.

Be Clear About What You Want

The question is how to sort out all the conflicting feelings. This comes down to (a) defining your objectives and being willing and able to redefine them as your child matures and (b) staying true to your objectives, even during a hotly contested game when you're surrounded by other parents screaming their heads off. This, of course, is the really hard part.

When your child is five, you may simply want her to have fun. When she's fifteen, you may be hoping that basketball will provide a boost with college admissions, or will keep her fit and help reduce the stress in her life. Or you may want your child to be the star of at least one high school team. But bear in mind that your objectives may be different from your child's. The *New York Times* published a survey in 1977 in which parents and kids (ages eight to ten) chose the three most important reasons for the child to play competitive sports. The parents chose "being challenged," "learning to compete," and "winning." The kids chose "having fun," "learning new skills," and "making friends." As I said before, being a sports parent is tough, and the job description keeps changing, so parents have to stay on their toes.

Clearly and above all, youth sports should be about having fun. This is particularly true in America, where our population is becoming progressively more inactive. Several teenage patients in my practice have burned out on their sport; they don't play anymore. What we are after is long-term health, and that means kids staying physically active their whole life. Good physical habits are established when kids are young, and if they aren't having fun, they don't keep playing.

As a parent you need to keep this fact in mind at all times. Sometimes it's hard, especially when you've been reduced to playing chauffeur most days. It sometimes helps to remember that you only have the kids at home for eighteen years, and then there are no more games to attend (unless you and they are very lucky, and they go to a nearby college and make the team).

And speaking of chauffeuring, remember this: When it comes to your kid's sports life, the only time you should be in the driver's seat is when you're taking him to his games.

Recently, an eleven-year-old three-sport athlete — tennis, soccer, and ice hockey — came to my office with an overuse knee injury that required surgery. Over the summer he practiced each sport two hours a day and went to a sports camp for each sport. During the school year, he had school team practice in the afternoon and practice for his club team at night. His mother proudly repeated, "He is the best player on the soccer team and the best player on the hockey team, the best." It was clear that his being the best was the only thing that mattered to her. My patient, on the other hand, never smiled, even when his mother reported his stats. He talked about his sports participation with not an iota of excitement or pleasure, as though sports were a form of servitude. I saw him as a victim of parental pressure, someone who because of his parents' personal needs had completely lost sight of the bigger picture of enjoyment as the reason to play sports. These parents' desire for reflected glory blinds them to what is best for their child in the long run.

Most parents want the best for their children. They want to make the world a better place for their children, and they want their children's life to be better than their own. Often accompanying this yearning for generational improvement, however, is a need for the child to redeem the failures of the parent, to avenge the parent for any remembered insult or slight, whether in high school, the workplace, or elsewhere.

When there's a mismatch between the parents' expectations and the child's talents, tension is likely to surface. The parent who desperately wants his kid to be a star can make a bench player miserable through overt or covert criticism. When the child is an athlete but the parent wants a pianist or dancer, she might belittle sports and the child's athletic abilities, and even manipulate schedules to interfere with team practices or games. Even when parents are careful to say little to their child about sports, the child often picks up on their deep-rooted interests (for example, the father is a volunteer coach and watches all the games he can on television) and tries to comply even when she has little talent and prefers other activities. With matching expectations, however, life is more pleasant.

Sports, parents, and children can be a volatile combination. I tell parents it's a good idea to step back and think calmly about a number of issues here:

- What do you really want your child to get from sports? What are your short-term goals? What are your long-term goals? Short-term goals might be to have fun, develop good social skills, make friends, enhance self-esteem. Long-term goals might include to develop athletic talent, to maintain fitness, to develop an identity unique to the child and separate from the parent, to develop lifelong habits of physical activity. *Note:* Throughout life, fitness is correlated with a reduced incidence of depression.
- Are your own hopes and expectations helping or hindering you from reaching your goals for your child?
- How might your experience with sports affect your relationship with your child? Will it bring you closer or push you apart?

Are You an Overinvolved Parent?

One way to think about overinvolvement is to consider where your emotional resources are invested. Financial advisers steer clients away from overinvestment in any one area. Yet every weekend we see vast numbers of financiers, not to mention doctors, lawyers, merchant chiefs, who have clearly overinvested emotionally in their children's athletic lives.

What exactly does that mean? And are you among this growing legion? Here's a quiz to help you figure out where you stand.

The Eleven Warning Signs of Emotional Overinvestment

Respond yes or no to the following:

1. You never miss your child's games, even if it means sneaking out of important business meetings.

2. Your entire social life revolves around your kid's team.

3. Your kid's performance and the team's fortunes are your primary topics of conversation.

4. You yell yourself hoarse at your kid's games.

5. You keep written records of your kid's performance (batting average, points per game). (Parents of high schoolers who are considering playing in college may be off the hook on this one. See Chapter 11.)

6. You let your athlete slack off on household chores because the games and practices are so demanding.

7. It's hard to talk comfortably with parents of players who are better than your child.

8. When your kid's team wins, you're elated; when they lose, you're depressed for the rest of the week.

9. Your child never smiles in your presence on game day, win or lose.

10. You're having sports-related arguments with your kid more than once a week.

11. Your kid complains to you directly that you need to back off.

If you responded yes to more than five of these statements, the diagnosis is clear: a case of emotional overinvestment.

The Consequences of Emotional Overinvestment

So what? you might ask. Why shouldn't I go to my kid's games? She's only going to play for a few years. What's so terrible about yelling myself hoarse? Isn't that the American way: rooting for the home team on Friday night? And up to a point, you would be right. If athletics is important to your child, of course you should take an interest. If she wants you at the games, try to arrange to be there. Dinner table conversations about the upcoming game or the new players on the team can constitute a healthy component of family life. And a certain amount of socializing with teammates' families is appropriate and pleasurable. But remember, "Moderation in all things." If your family discusses only sports and never touches on political events, or books or movies, history or science, you're overly focused on sports and likely to be shortchanging your kids. These are the years when you want to be introducing your children to the wider world and developing their curiosity. Your obsession with sports can stunt your kids' intellectual, emotional, and social growth, leaving them less than fully rounded. And if their interest in sports wanes, or if they sustain a long-term injury that prevents their involvement, it may be extremely difficult for them to find other fruitful and satisfying outlets.

Basically, your involvement with your kid's athletic activity verges on overinvolvement when it adversely affects your child. The last three warning signs relate to your child's mental state and his relationship with you. If he no longer seems to be happy playing, if sports have become a frequent flashpoint in your family, if your child expressly tells you he's unhappy with your behavior at the games or your attitude toward sports, you probably have some real soul-searching to do.

As we've seen, one of the main benefits of youth sports is the satisfaction and joy they produce for the players. Serious athletes, especially as they reach high school age, spend long hours honing their skills and working with their coach and teammates on tactics and techniques. The payoff for all this hard work is the satisfaction they derive from improving as players, being part of a team, becoming fitter and healthier, and, we hope, winning with enough frequency to reinforce the other benefits. In addition, sports should be a source of sheer fun as the young athlete experiences the unique pleasure of performing at peak capacity, preferably with teammates she likes and respects, under a coach she admires. When you overinvest in your kid's athletics, you create a drag on the benefits your child would otherwise derive and produce unnecessary stress in her life. And no child or adolescent needs extra stress.

Diversify Your Emotional Portfolio

So what to do if you flunked the overinvestment quiz? Diversify. You can probably figure out your own cures to suit your particular family configuration, but here are some things to try:

The Rule of Three

If your child says you're overinvolved or that she doesn't want you at her games, try skipping every third game. When Game Day No. 3 arrives, say to your kid, "Good-bye, have fun, play well, and good luck." Then, to ease the withdrawal, treat yourself to a movie or brunch with friends. In time this painful ritual may become easier, even pleasurable. You'll catch up with films you've missed because you were on the sidelines and rediscover the pleasures of Sunday eggs benedict, which you probably haven't had since your child was born.

Avocational Therapy

Take up new leisure-time activities of your own. You and your spouse can enroll in that ballroom dancing class you've been promising yourselves. Or pull out the darkroom equipment that's been gathering dust in your attic since your kid started playing sports. Or you can volunteer to be a ref — for other kids' teams.

Start Your Own Team

Instead of living vicariously through your child, take up his sport yourself. Form a team of like-minded adults. I know of a group of soccer moms who did just that. When their daughters were eleven and starting to play soccer seriously, some of the mothers had the self-awareness to realize they were jealous. Their kids were doing what they never did: playing a sport they loved seriously and regularly. These mothers formed a team called (what else?) the Soccer Moms. Some had never played before, but they trained, recruited a handful of younger, more experienced players, hired a coach, and joined a league. Five years later they're still going strong, and have even played in a tournament in Ireland!

The Sports Parent's Mantra

If you still find you're living vicariously through your child's athletic life, do the following: Before going to your child's game, look yourself in the mirror, take a deep cleansing breath, and say, "I'm not

Johnny, Johnny's not me." Repeat this as necessary with your own child's name until you know you no longer need "Johnny" to make up for all the injustices in your own life.

Supporting Your Child

Now that you've gotten a handle on your own issues and have attained a near-perfect zen state of sports parenthood, it's time to focus on how, in this newly enlightened spirit, you can best support your child and the team.

One major, perennial, and difficult parenting issue (and not just for sports) is how to encourage high standards without pressuring too much. How do we balance pushing/coaxing our child to reach new, fulfilling achievements against nurturing what he can and wants to do? This primarily means paying close attention to the child's patterns of behavior and response. Does Julia eagerly embrace new experiences (and if so, does this entail excessive risk-taking?), or does she stand back and evaluate the situation before dipping a toe in the water (and if so, is she overly fearful?)? Is Tom clear about what he wants (for example, an electric guitar), or does he want to try something new every week (the guitar, then tae kwon do, then chess)? Does Robert tend to overestimate his abilities and performance, thus leading to repeated disappointment, or does he underestimate them, thus avoiding challenge and new experiences? Or does he usually evaluate them objectively?

Parents also need to figure out what evidence is relevant. Is a particular incident or remark a blip or a trend? If your child suddenly doesn't want to play, you need to analyze whether she's entered a new phase of development — perhaps theater has become more compelling — or whether someone has been mean ("When are you going to learn to kick the ball?") or whether her reluctance is an expression of momentary insecurity, but she'd actually like to continue playing. Blip versus trend is always a difficult call, even for the most observant parents, especially because children are often simply unable to explain their decisions. Parents have to listen and watch for any scraps of evidence to guide them.

One useful strategy is to help your child focus on parts of the game where he can exert himself (such as positioning, decision-making, skills). Remind him that there's nothing he can do about some things (field conditions, the referee, the weather), and that complaining about these elements will simply distract him from playing his best. You can discuss the differences with your child; you can also set an example by cheering for good plays and good decisions ("Good idea!") and being calm about bad calls by the officials (say nothing, or if you must, say something like "Yes, that was a bad call, but it's part of the game").

Another strategy that works well is to help your child set attainable, legitimate goals (such as "Remember to look up when you have the ball," "See if you can shoot ten times during the game," "Just do your best, so that you're proud of your effort"). Listen to what your child wants to do. If he doesn't want to play, don't make him — unless your repeated experience is that he needs to be coaxed. Talk about the feelings of failure as well as success. It's important for kids to learn to handle losing and failing, just as it's important to learn about winning. They should strive to win, but not at the expense of having fun. In general, girls seem better at enjoying the experience of playing than boys, who tend to be raised to win.

In a series of school squash matches, a young friend named Sasha always lost to Malina, never scoring more than four points. Sasha was anxious and unhappy the night before the final match. Her parents suggested that she try to score six points this time. The next day Sasha came home beaming: She had scored *eight* points against Malina! She had still lost the match, but she was a winner in her own mind because she had achieved the goal she wanted to.

An added wrinkle to the difficulty of balancing high expectations with low pressure is that boys and girls often respond differently to pressure and criticism. Most boys seem able to take them in stride, whereas girls are often exceptionally sensitive to what they perceive as criticism. As one father put it, "Girls seem to wear their skin inside out."

With both boys and girls, however, positive reinforcement is always better than a negative approach. In one exercise, basketball players were divided into two groups. One group analyzed films of free throws they had made; the other analyzed films of free throws missed. The group shown the made shots did far better in the next game they played. Positive reinforcement is the better tool for a variety of possible reasons, among them stimulating the visual memory of having been successful and building greater self-confidence.

But even when parents think they're being positive, girls often hear the most innocuous statement as pressure and respond with fury. If a parent says, "Did you practice dribbling today?" the girl hears — usually correctly — "You need to work on your dribbling." "You forgot to practice, didn't you?" may lead to nuclear holocaust in your kitchen. Try to think in terms of positive reinforcement and give up on the concept of constructive criticism. In the minds of children, who are always at the mercy of their all-powerful parents, there is no such thing as constructive criticism. One useful mantra for parents is: "Do I want to be right, or do I want to be effective?" Indeed, this mantra can prove invaluable in a wide variety of parenting and social situations, sports-related or not.

One major source of difficulty between parents and children is that parents know how much they could improve their children's lives by sharing their own hard-earned wisdom ("Reread your essay before handing it in"; "If you always put your glove in the same place, you won't waste time looking for it"). Children, however, all too often intransigently reject parental advice and must discover how to manage in the world through their own experience. And "experience" more often than not refers to bad decisions recollected in tranquillity. It's hard for parents to see their children heading for mistakes, but unless they risk serious injury, it's usually better to let them figure out what to do by themselves. If you're lucky, when they fail they'll come to you for advice and might even act on what you tell them.

If your child asks for advice, offer it humbly and give yourself credit for establishing this type of relationship with him. But otherwise, remember that one of the most frustrating aspects of parenthood is knowing that your experience could save your child vast amounts of time, pain, and suffering but finding that he not only doesn't want to take your advice, he doesn't even want to hear it.

If you cannot resist offering advice, couching it positively is usually more effective than putting it negatively. Try saying "Remember to take your cleats" instead of "Don't forget your cleats." "Remember" is a suggestion; "Don't forget" is nagging, because the wording assumes the child will forget or has forgotten. (However, if you repeat "Remember" often enough, that terminology, too, will become nagging, because it's automatic, and thus it will also be resented.)

If you think the child's negligence is serious enough, you can take a stringent approach with severe consequences. One exasperated mother let her child show up for a soccer tournament without her shoes.

Child: Mom, where are my cleats?
Mom: Under the stairs, right where I told you.
Child: [*Stunned silence, then loud penetrating wail.*]

With "tough love," the question is whether the punishment fits the crime.

It's really, really hard to strike a balance between restraint and action with a child who is working on being independent and self-reliant. I tell parents, Do your best and remember that nobody's perfect.

Some Specific Challenges

When I give talks about sports medicine around the country, parents always ask a lot of questions. And as an athlete myself, I've heard a lot of parent discussions on the sidelines. Below are some of the questions that come up over and over again.

Stress
My daughter gets nervous and sometimes even throws up before a big game. What should I do?

This is stress you and your child need to deal with. First consider whether you are contributing to her state of mind: How do you support her? Many parents, attempting to fulfill their parental responsibilities, try to improve a child's skills through constant "constructive" criticism of her playing, or offer "suggestions" that in fact make her feel less adequate. When a child complains or worries, especially one who is evidently under great stress, it's helpful simply to nod and agree sympathetically and *wait* to be asked for advice. And to hold your tongue if you aren't asked. (Of course, this is much easier said than done.)

One suggestion you might make right before a big event is to have her focus on a specific task at hand. Instead of her thinking "This is for the league championship," have her think "I need to stay with my mark," "I want to stay calm," or "I'm going to use a bounce pass more." This is the basis of mental toughness. It's also the way for the kid to not freeze up when she's on the foul line and to be able to score the go-ahead points at the end of the game.

Too Much Competitiveness
I see Little League parents constantly working their laptops and Palm Pilots at games so they can show the stats to their kids afterward. Is this focus on competitiveness okay?

In some areas, I think that the youth sports environment has spun out of control. In many areas of the country, adults have made the competition too serious for kids, especially the young ones.

As far as producing instant stats, I'd say it depends on the kids. If they view instant stats as a parental idiosyncrasy irrelevant to their lives, it's fine. If the constant calculation makes them feel pressure and have less fun playing, it's not.

The essence of sports is organized competition (I win, you lose). One key to a satisfying sports experience for your child is to make sure she's playing at the right level of competition: enough to challenge her to learn more and work harder, but not so much that she feels hopeless about improving and depressed about losing all the time. This is true for athletes at all ages (and for nonsports activities as well). Competition is not a bad thing. It's a part of life, and learning to understand and deal with it is not only healthy, it is also necessary to adult success.

Most kids enjoy playing in rec leagues where "everyone plays," at least until the fourth or fifth grade. At that point, they tend to self-select — the ones who want more competition try out for travel teams, the ones who just want to play stay in the rec leagues. This is the age when kids start the long process of figuring out what they're interested in and good at. Self-selection in sports is one element of that process, and something to be encouraged. Every kid really is different, and no one formula is true for everyone. Do not apply your own sports memories (whether miserable or glorious) to your child's life, but help him pursue what *he* wants. Listen to what he says, and pay attention to his behavior.

Kids who play individual sports (tennis, skating, gymnastics) may seek out competition earlier, maybe in third grade or fourth grade. Parents should be sure to try to balance the sports with noncompetitive activities such as classes in art, music, or theater. Otherwise kids may burn out early or grow up to be too competitive and stressed, working for straight A's, striving for wins all the time, and having less fun in too many areas of their lives.

For both team players and individual athletes, the signs of excessive competition are subtle. Be attentive to the following behavior:

- Feigning injury
- Resisting attending practice
- Fear of games (or lack of enthusiasm)
- Somatic complaints (stomachache, headache)

Keep in mind that the long-term goal for your child is the development of good physical and mental habits, generally manifested as

- Athletic participation across the lifespan.
- Balance between hard work and enjoyment.
- Productive participation in the larger community.

Tryouts

How can I help my child with tryouts?

The short answer is "Stay away." By the time your child is ready for selective sports, he's ready to deal with competitive tryouts. He should know to:

- Be in shape (your child should start conditioning programs, both weights and endurance, four to six weeks before the sports season).
- Practice his skills regularly.
- Eat properly.
- Get a good night's sleep for the two nights beforehand.
- Demonstrate what he can do.
- Be friendly and respectful to the adults in charge.

Your job is to complete the paperwork and write the check. Period. You can't hover in the vicinity during an algebra or Latin test — the same goes for tryouts. Enlightened leagues keep parents away to reduce inappropriate interference and the athletes' stress.

The long answer: Do all of the above and more. We have all seen how politics can deform what should be a purely democratic, merit-based experience for children. Politics includes everything from the coach's favoring his own child to the wealthy parent who is willing to subsidize a whole team (paying for uniforms, tournament fees, transportation, a trainer) in order for his less-qualified child to play.

Even if your kid has demonstrated superior athletic talent, it's a good idea to get involved with the organization and get to know the club officials, the coaches, the parents whose children are acknowledged as dominant players. Make yourself useful. Volunteer your time to do whatever the league needs, whether it's sweeping leaves off the tennis courts, picking up broken glass from urban playing fields, developing and administering insurance policies, or helping to construct the schedule of games.

Whether we like it or not, the rule of "It's not *what* you know, it's *who* you know" holds true in children's sports as well as in the world of business. If you have a legitimate complaint or suggestion about tryouts or anything else, the decision-makers are more likely to go out of their way to listen and act if they know you; know they can count on you to be level-headed, objective, and resourceful; know that you will help out when needed; know that you care about the game and the children involved, and are not simply a rabid partisan interested only in advancing the career of your own offspring.

Furthermore, contributing time and energy will (a) tell many children that they are important, (b) help their teams and division run more smoothly, and (c) convey the valuable lesson that "all politics are local," or that knowing more people is better than knowing few people.

Some competitive clubs have mandated that teams have professional coaches instead of parent volunteers, and that tryouts be supervised by independent observers to minimize parent manipulation of teams. These rules are a good idea but, given the energy, ingenuity, and duplicity of parents desperate to give their children an advantage, they are not foolproof. Nothing is.

Quitting the Team
My child wants to stop playing. If I let her quit, won't I be teaching her that commitment and responsibility don't count?

The important questions are:

- What is it that my child doesn't want to play — is it the sport, the team, the type of team (competitive versus recreational)?
- What are the pros and cons of playing or not playing?
- How will it affect her team?
- Why does my child not want to play?
- Why do I want my child to play?

One mother told me that her eighth-grader, Sandra, wanted to quit school basketball midseason because a clique of "popular" girls on the team excluded her and never passed to her. Sandra had already brought it up to the coach, who spoke to the girls in question, but nothing seemed to change.

We all know girls that age can be ingeniously nasty. I asked the mother how much Sandra wanted to play basketball. If she's lukewarm and the unpleasant court atmosphere turns her off, maybe she can swim or run cross-country instead. On the other hand, if she loves basketball and is devastated by the situation, the mother needs to intervene in some way.

I told her to attend as many games as possible to see for herself what was going on. Maybe she would notice specific behaviors or moments, on the part of Sandra as well as the team, and be able to make suggestions to her daughter or the coach. Maybe the girls aren't passing to her because they don't look up and have no idea where anybody is on the court. That would be annoying, but it's different from cliquishness.

I also suggested that the mother talk to the coach herself, and if that was unsatisfactory, to the athletic director. In addition, she might point out to Sandra that (a) next year will be completely different because the team makeup will change, and (b) if she quits midseason, she'll lose a lot of practice time and not be as good next year.

The mother should also ask Sandra what she'd like her to do, or what Sandra thinks she herself could do to change the situation. If she really loves basketball, she should stick with it unless the situation is completely unbearable. She should also sign up for an out-of-school league: she would get to play more, improve her skills, meet new girls, and have a good time.

How you respond to your child's wanting to quit will depend to some extent on the age of the child. If the problem involves a team sport, you should consider how much obligation your child owes the team and what kind of lesson you will impart if you allow her to stop playing.

The Younger Child (5–11): If the child is just starting out, he may be confused about the rules of the game or be scared of getting hurt. You can explain the rules and demonstrate what it's like to be hit by the ball — which isn't as bad as most kids think. You can also practice skills with him so he feels more comfortable with the game.

If your child is adamant about stopping and has tried participating for two or three weeks, let her stop. At this age, the obligation to a team is minimal; one player's dropping off is unlikely to make a significant difference in the experience of the other children.

The Older Child (12–18): With a child who has previously been committed to sports, a dramatic change in interests should be looked into. The issues are complicated. Why does she want to stop? Find out if she feels she's hit a wall and cannot improve further. Does she feel she cannot live up to the expectations of her peers and the adults around her? Does she feel overwhelmed by demands on her time? These are serious and valid reasons to stop.

However, these reasons must also be balanced against the long-term benefits of continuing to play (staying fit, understanding teamsmanship, learning to weather rough times and emerge from a slump). Could this be a temporary phase that, if played through, will end? Will she feel that she quit something she loves doing because of what other people think? There is also the issue of her obligations and commitments to others if she plays on a team. How much does her team depend on her showing up and playing hard, or sitting on the bench and being subbed in? If a competitive team has chosen your child over others for a limited number of roster spots, dropping out is likely to severely hamper their game. Is she willing to finish out the season?

If you allow your child to quit during the season, you might be encouraging her to give up quickly in the face of other challenges. In addition, the perceived message might be that your child's needs or wants are paramount and that those of others don't count.

Maria was a stellar young soccer player who could defend her goal against all comers, distribute the ball to the midfield and forwards, and score when put up front. She had never played basketball before, but she made her school's JV team because very few of her classmates tried out that year. She couldn't catch the ball or throw it accurately, and set picks on her own teammates because she didn't understand the game. Whenever she was subbed in, it was generally worth at least four points to their opponents.

Midway through the season, Maria wanted to drop off the basketball team. Many of her teammates, while recognizing her weaknesses, believed that a commitment is absolute and that dropping off was "unworthy." (This is a typical adolescent response; teens have difficulty with nuance and shades of gray. It's much easier to embrace a rule and stick to it through thick and thin.) The coach, too, thought the girl should honor her commitment, although he did not offer her extra practice or even a hope of more playing time.

Various parents suggested that in this case the goals of playing on a team, other than honoring commitment, were not being

met: Maria had shown no talent for this game and was not learning any new skills, nor was she likely to. She was given little
playing time and complained about this even though she knew
she didn't deserve more minutes. She felt bad about herself and
her contribution to the team. There seemed little reason for her
to remain on the team. She wouldn't be contributing to her own
growth or to the growth of the team.

I agree with the parents. Whatever the decision, however, the
main thing, for both parents and the athlete, is that the child be
clear about her reasons, either for staying or for leaving the
team. And those reasons should take into account the consequences for her teammates and not just herself.

Being Cut
What if my child doesn't make the team?
Be very sympathetic. It's always painful, for both parent and
child, when the child fails to achieve something he really wants.
With sports, the pain of this failure is magnified because it is
very public, and it also entails a lack of access to a particular
social network, which can be inordinately important in the eyes
of adolescents.

Depending on your relationship, you might say to your child:
"Can you look yourself in the eye and tell yourself honestly that
you did everything you could to prepare for this tryout? If you
did everything possible, at least you have the satisfaction of
knowing that you made a genuine commitment to something
you care about, and you should keep trying to improve your performance. I know this doesn't help now, but when you're older it
might."

It's extremely helpful for you and your child to assess her
chances beforehand. Who else is likely to be trying out? How
many will be chosen? What is the coach looking for? What are
your child's strengths and weaknesses? Help your athlete to be
objective when answering these questions and to develop realis-
tic expectations. That way, she is freer to do her best without

crushing pressure and to be able to use the tryout as a learning experience.

If your child loves this particular sport, do encourage him to practice and to play on other teams. With practice and play he can improve his skills, and with age his body will change. Not making the team one year doesn't mean he can't make it the next.

It does not help the situation or your child's maturation if you rant about the unfairness of the process, how the coaches are biased, how the team is made up of friends of the manager, and so on. Set a good example for your child. Your child needs to deal with the disappointment and public humiliation and move on.

Later, when the pain has subsided, perhaps you can encourage your child to take up an entirely different sport, perhaps one better suited to his body type. For example, a tall slender player would probably fare better at basketball than at football.

Supporting the Team

When you sign your kid up for a team sport, you automatically take on certain responsibilities, not only to your child but also to the team. These responsibilities include pitching in to help the team function more smoothly. Sometimes clichés are true: There's no *I* in *team*, and teams work only when all the things that need to be done get done, such as driving for the carpool or sitting at the security desk at the local school for weekend basketball games.

Some Basics

Be respectful to all participants — your child's teammates, the opposing players, their parents, the coach, the officials. Assume they're doing their best, even when you can't figure out why they're doing what they're doing. Giving others the benefit of the doubt includes:

- Not *publicly* questioning (or sneering at) the lineup — especially when your own child doesn't start or get the position he wants.
- Not groaning audibly at a missed shot.
- Not shouting instructions to your child (or other players) — it just confuses them to hear multiple directions.
- Not criticizing the officials.

Learn the rules of the game. Every sport has many rules, and some are complicated. In addition, the question almost always arises of when to apply the rules: When is a decision clear-cut and when is it a judgment call? With younger children (say, under nine), when is it better to enforce the rules and when is it better to let them play on?

Pop Quiz

Can a soccer ref card a player who taunts or threatens an opponent after a game?

When can high school basketball players enter the lane after a foul shot?

Can a football score be 1–0?

Answers

The soccer ref is in authority from the moment the team sets foot on the field until the players leave at the end of the game.

It depends on the league. In many leagues, boys can step into the lane when the ball hits the rim, girls when the ball is released.

The score for a football game is recorded as 1–0 if one team forfeits.

- Knowing the rules will help you stop screaming at the officials.
- You can use your knowledge to explain to others — players and parents — what the officials are ruling and why.
- If poor officiating is affecting game results, you can write up evaluation reports for the sponsoring league. If there is no system of evaluation reports, you can volunteer to set one up.

Pretend your own child is not playing and act accordingly. That is, try to be dispassionate — at least once in a while — and enjoy the game for its ebb and flow, the strategy, the skills, individualism, creativity, intelligence, and common purpose of all the players, rather than focusing on your own child's performance.

Fulfill your obligations:
- Be on time (for practice, games, meetings); wasting other people's time by making them wait is selfish and disrespectful.
- Do what you say you'll do, so others can plan for the good of the whole team.
- Recognize that in order for the team to function, parents must pitch in and help. Signing your kid up means obligations for the parents.

Extra credit:
- Cheer for the opponents when they do something well.
- Set a limit on the number of times you yell your child's name per game (say, five times, always communicating something positive, of course), and make sure to praise the other players more than you do your own.
- Do something special for your child's team at least once during the season (organize a bake sale, plan an awards banquet).
- Congratulate the coach and players after a win. Commiserate after a loss without recriminations ("We just couldn't catch a break," *not* "If only Jason hadn't lost his man" or "Hometown ref").

When you're watching your children play an organized sport, the main thing to remember is how you want them to remember you when they are parents themselves. As supportive, enthusiastic, generous, and fair? As out of control, abusive, win-at-all-costs? It's easy to get excited when you see kids demonstrating their abilities. But it's also important not to get overexcited and demand something the kids don't want or can't achieve: victory above all, and outstanding

Threats to the Players

On rare occasions, a parent gets so caught up in youth games and is so desperate to win that he resorts to violence and threats. Adults have been known to say to kids, softly, so they won't be overheard, things like "If you come near the sideline again, I'll kill you." This is harassment or menacing, depending on how threatened the player feels, and both are illegal. Players should know that if they ever feel physically threatened, they can tell their coach or the official, who should summon the police immediately. This is what cell phones were invented for. Even if the adult denies threatening anyone, other parents will now be keeping an eye on him. Thankfully, these measures are seldom called for, but kids and parents need to know they have recourse if someone gets out of hand.

individual performance. It's *their* game, not yours. Let them have fun. Stop interfering and allow them to grow up to be autonomous, confident, reality-based individuals.

And surely it goes without saying that parents should never bring alcohol to games.

The Box Score

- Be clear about your own issues, find a good balance, and make sure you're involved, but not overinvolved.
- Recognize the warning signs of when sports become too serious in your family.
- Find out what your child wants and needs and help him attain his goals.
- Help the team and the league in appropriate ways.
- At all times set a good example. Be courteous and respectful to all participants — players, coaches, officials.

Chapter 3

Put Me In, Coach

WORKING WITH THE COACH

This chapter covers the hallmarks of good coaching and what to do if you or your child is unhappy with the coach.

Coaching is demanding and stressful. Whether he's a former All-American in a high-profile high school program or a first-time volunteer parent in a rec league, when the team isn't winning, the coach gets blamed. Even when the team is winning, complaints can bubble up — about starting, about playing time, about position assignments, about tactics, about any number of things — because coaching is something everyone thinks they can do better than the guy (or gal) who's doing it.

Great coaches not only know the game (skills and tactics), but also have the knack of bringing out the best in young players, on the field and off. By the time an athlete reaches middle school or high school, she probably spends more time with her coach than with any adult other than her parents. Besides learning rules, strategies, and skills, what kids learn from sports is values. They learn to care about good sportsmanship as well as winning, to balance cooperation with competitiveness, to appreciate effort as well as results, and to understand the importance of a positive, confident attitude. They also learn that they can improve their play through practice, and that they have control over this process. They learn these values from the grownups around them — their parents and their coaches. In many ways, the tasks of all these adults are the same: to set a good example and keep things in perspective. The coach, however, can often get kids to work harder than their parents can. First of all, because sports are inherently important to athletes, they're predisposed to listen to the coach. Second, the coach is not a parent and thus is unencumbered by the emotional baggage of that relationship. Third, the coach has one focused area through which to teach kids — sports — whereas parents have to teach children to improve their math skills, write thank-you notes, and take out the garbage, a muddle in which clear messages can get lost.

The role of the coach changes as kids grow older. The skills and strategies become more sophisticated; the players' understanding of the game as well as their own responsibilities to the team increase. Finally, the stakes get higher as the players start to apply to colleges. No matter what the players' age, however, one constant obtains: Coaches must be able to teach.

Coaches come in two varieties: parent or community volunteers and paid professionals. Recreational and youth league teams, especially for younger players, are typically coached by intrepid dads or moms, who may or may not know and love the sport in question, but sign up out of a sense of responsibility and commitment to their kids and the community. School teams are almost always run by teachers or coaches engaged or assigned by the athletic department. There seems to be an increasing trend for club teams, especially those for older players, to hire professionals as well. Parents might think about hiring a team coach the way they think about hiring a piano teacher. The kids deserve to work with someone who can teach them more than volunteers can. This is especially true with those sports such as water polo and lacrosse that moms and dads generally didn't play as kids. Coaches of these kinds of teams are hired either by the team parents or by a sponsoring organization (church, community center) or league.

Both types have advantages and drawbacks. First there are the bottom-line issues. Parents or sponsors may not be willing or able to foot the bill for a professional coach. Volunteers come at the low, low price of free, but sometimes the old adage "You get what you pay for" rings all too true. In my experience, by and large, volunteer coaches do an outstanding job, but of course, there are egregious exceptions.

Sometimes, for example, parents who are volunteer coaches favor their own kids in flagrant ways such as giving them preferential playing time and position assignments, appointing them as captain of the team, and giving them the postseason awards, such as MVP. This, of course, infuriates the other parents, but unless they act in concert, there's generally little they can do. (It's like school, when parents try to oust a really bad teacher.) The parents' success in these cases depends on having a league or club head who is interested in broad issues of fairness, or at least a mission statement articulating some ideal of good sportsmanship and offering an opportunity to every player to excel. When parents find themselves up against a coach who is interested only in the advancement of his own children, they must seek support from others, or decide whether the benefits of staying are worth it.

Because they're being paid, professional coaches can arguably be held to a higher level of accountability with respect to questions of equity as well as to issues relating to player development and team success. It's easier to deal with disparities in playing time when the players involved are not the coach's kids (though it's never all that easy in any circumstances!). And there's a justifiable assumption that the professional coach's expertise will result in the individual players and the team as whole improving over time, which can be more readily discussed and addressed as necessary if the coach is an employee.

Volunteer Coaches

Some 2.5 million adults volunteer annually to coach youth sports teams, and of those, about 60 percent coach their own kids. This is a generous service to the community and to the children.

Rec leagues are always looking for volunteer coaches. Don't worry if you know little about the game. To stay ahead of the kids, read the rulebook, watch games on television, and look around and do what other coaches are doing with their teams.

What all children need — at five, at fifteen — is to spend time in the company of a grownup who cares about them as human beings, who is interested in their progress (no matter how small or large), and who habitually responds to life with intellectual curiosity, confidence, common sense, and a sense of proportion. You can do all of these things without knowing the game, and you will learn about the game as you and the children go along. Many respected long-time coaches knew nothing when they began to coach, having taken on the job only because they were told "You have to coach or there won't be a team."

But there are a couple of big "ifs." Volunteer only if you're willing to show up for every game and every practice (well, maybe one absence per season), and if you feel you can be fair to all players, even the ones who prefer picking daisies to keeping their eye on the ball.

Your behavior sets an example for the children and the other parents. This means they will all observe your treatment (whether respectful or disrespectful, consistent or inconsistent) of players, parents, and officials, your willingness to spend time with the children and teach them skills, your reliability in keeping promises (to show up, to leave the worst hitter in the lineup when you most need a hit). They will also observe your sportsmanship. Do you applaud good plays made by the opposing team? In a situation mentioned earlier, do you inform the ref of an opponent's goal if the referee didn't see it, even if it means facing the wrath of the team parents and possibly losing the game? (I believe the answer depends on the age of the children: The younger they are, the more necessary it is for the coach to speak up and teach the team that winning due to an officiating error is neither satisfying nor something to be proud of. When they're older, however, and winning becomes more important, you and the team have no obligation to make victory more difficult for yourselves by being proactively scrupulous. But of course you can speak up if you think circumstances warrant it.)

Think about how you'll feel about your coaching ten years later. Will you be pleased with yourself and will your child? Or will you be ashamed? An older friend of mine who coached his daughter's Little League team once manipulated the lineup during an important game to work in a good hitter. Years later, he says he still remembers the look of pain and disappointment on the child he moved back, and has always regretted his decision.

I'm a coach, and my child thinks I should pay more attention to her than to the other kids.

This is a widespread problem for young kids, and it might help to point that out to your child. Coaches need to appear objective and concerned about the good of the whole team. As they grow older, kids with parents in positions of authority have a more sophisticated worry: that parents striving not to show favoritism are harder on their own children than on their teammates. You, perhaps in conjunction with your child, have to decide whether the stress is too severe to justify your continuing to coach your kid's team. You could coach another team, but bear in mind that this will cause scheduling difficulties if you want to see your own child play. (These issues also come up for refs.)

When should I stop being the coach?

When you can no longer help the kids improve their skills or devise winning team strategies for them, it's time to turn in your clipboard. Pick up a whistle and volunteer to officiate, starting with games for younger children. This means learning every rule and discovering how incredibly difficult it is to see everything that happens all the time and make instant decisions about what is an infraction and what isn't. With young kids, you will also have to decide how much to teach as you officiate, and how much latitude to allow in order to let them keep playing. It's a very hard job and seldom appreciated, but officiating will make you a more knowledgeable sports parent as well as a good citizen.

Training for Volunteer Coaches

Those stalwart, often heroic, parents or other interested members of the community who volunteer to coach almost always need training. Indeed, anyone who works with groups of kids needs training in communications, child development, and age-appropriate content. Athletic coaches in particular, who spend many hours with their charges, must learn how to effectively use the great power they possess.

Besides sports-specific fundamentals, training for volunteer coaches should cover:

- Communication and teaching
- Child development (physical and psychological)
- Fitness
- Sportsmanship
- Cooperation
- Nonviolent conflict resolution
- Basic first aid

These topics are essential because sports involve the whole person. Leagues can offer beginning, intermediate, and advanced levels of training, rather than a one-size-fits-all course for its volunteers.

The basic premise in training a coach is that coaching is teaching, and the coach must be prepared to teach not just skills and strategies, but also ethics, motivation, and long-term respect for the game and oneself.

If the league your child plays in doesn't have a training program for its coaches, figure out a way to set one up. A key component of such a program is assessment. Once trained, coaches should be observed and evaluated by league officials. At the end of each season, parents (especially of younger players) should be asked to complete questionnaires addressing the coach's strengths and weaknesses.

Positive Coaching

The Positive Coaching Alliance, a not-for-profit organization based at Stanford University, runs workshops that teach coaches how to improve individual and team performance through its "positive coaching" mental model. Its mission is to "transform youth sports so that sports can transform youth." Among its many practical ideas about how to teach and motivate kids are its exhortation to redefine "winner" as someone who gets back up after a loss and tries harder, and a technique called "positive charting," which is a quantified method of giving feedback.

Assessing the Coach

How do you know when the coach is doing a good job? This will depend on your team's goals, which in turn are partly dependent on the age of the players.

Again, with younger kids, coaches should be expected to ensure the players are having fun, teach them good values (such as sportsmanship), instill a love of the game, and impart basic rules, skills, and age-appropriate tactics. For beginners (say, ages five to eight or nine), I subscribe wholeheartedly to the egalitarian philosophy of organizations like the American Youth Soccer Organization. Everyone on the team should get roughly the same amount of playing time, there should be no bench — everyone should be able to start some of the time, and everyone should have a turn at every position (no sticking the worst athlete exclusively in right field). The coach needs to bend over backward to be fair to everyone.

Positive coaching has been proven effective with every age group. With young players it's a must. Virtually everything out of the coach's mouth should be "Good job!," "Good idea!," "Nice try!," "Better luck next time!" Even corrective advice should be expressed positively, in terms of what the player should do in the future, such as "Next time try being more aggressive at the plate; take your cuts" — not "Don't stand there with your bat on your shoulder!" or "Try bending your knees more when you're taking a foul shot" — not "Don't shoot flatfooted!"

An individual with a good understanding of developmental psychology and an ability to manage young groups will be more effective with novice athletes than a more knowledgeable, experienced coach without such skills. Warmth, friendliness, enthusiasm, combined with an ability to give direction calmly and clearly are essential attributes in working with this age group, more so than a sophisticated understanding of the game. Indeed, I've often seen coaches who have grown up playing a sport become frustrated and even angry when dealing with the inevitable ineptitude of beginners. It's better to have a parent-volunteer coach who is a novice at the sport but empathetic with the kids than a high-powered expert who can't deal with young players' lack of skill and inability to focus.

As young athletes grow older, team goals change. Winning becomes much more important. To succeed in a competitive situation, players need to refine their skills and learn the nuances of the game. They must commit to a demanding work ethic and to giving their all. In team sports, they must learn to play and behave unselfishly, subordinating their own individual desires (starting,

Name That Team

I recently observed a twenty-something former soccer player who had volunteered to coach a team of nine-year-old girls brilliantly solve one of the thorniest problems in all of youth sports: naming the team. After he painfully elicited a few suggestions from the girls, it came time to vote. But no one dared raise a hand for any of the proposed names for fear of being scorned and derided for liking something the others did not. (Fear of being different reigns supreme at this age!) So this young coach had all the girls face outward in a circle and then called for a vote. This secret ballot resulted in an instantaneous decision. And thus were born the Red Foxes, who, by the way, went on to win the division championship, a result at least in part attributable to the young volunteer's understanding of both the game and the psyches of his young charges, and his ability to improvise.

getting more minutes, playing a favorite position, hogging the ball, and so on) in order to ensure the team's success. They also tend to specialize: they become offensive linemen or point guards or pitchers or wing midfielders, each position requiring particular skills and techniques. On older teams, playing time is generally expected to be allocated based on productivity, not equity. And older players (and their families) may want to showcase their abilities to help their college prospects. Clearly, playing on a high-school-age team with serious aspirations is a serious business, rife with potential for conflict. And the center of it all is the coach.

So coaching an older team becomes far more complicated and demanding, but the basic principles and the desirable attributes remain constant. No matter what age group or what kind of team she's working with, a good coach must be able to:

- Teach the rules, skills, and tactics of the game.
- Motivate the players to do their best and improve.

- Instill team spirit and a sense of working together for the common good.
- Teach respect for the game and other players (sportsmanship).

If you find a coach gifted in all four areas, consider yourself extremely lucky and be properly appreciative of this paragon. Praise him and (in the case of a club team) do all you can to make his life easier: volunteer to do the team paperwork, make all the arrangements for travel and uniforms, so that all he deals with is coaching.

What will you settle for? The most important element will depend on your objective: improvement? winning? learning new skills? fun? A coach needs some ability in all four areas. A complete washout in any one decreases the value of the other abilities. (However, as I suggested above, a coach who has great technical skills but has difficulty communicating is not a good match with young kids but may be acceptable for more experienced players, particularly as a skills trainer.)

How can you tell what you've got? This may be harder to evaluate than you think, especially if you're not around at practices or all the games (and as noted in Chapter 2, in general you should keep your distance, especially with older teams). But you can pretty much rest assured that the coach is doing okay if:

- The team wins a reasonable number of games (especially for older teams).
- The players are happy.
- They like going to games/practice.
- They respect the coach and speak well of him.
- They understand that effort is what's important.
- They are growing as players.
- The coach seems fair.

Some individuals go beyond normal coaching duties. One local figure skating coach attends my seminars and workshops to learn everything he can to keep his skaters healthy and strong. If one of his kids is injured, he accompanies the skater's family to my office for the exam. It is clear to his skaters, their parents, and to me that what he cares about most is the total well-being of his students. Both the kids and the parents trust him.

A Rewarding Game

A friend of mine is the volunteer coach of his twelve-year-old daughter's recreational soccer team. One day, toward the end of the season, many players were absent on game day (it was a heavy vacation and birthday weekend), and among the missing were the three strongest players. The coach told the team he didn't care what the result was, he just wanted to see them playing their best and playing hard. However, he added, if they wanted to borrow a few players from other teams who were waiting for the next games, he could easily arrange that. He was proud when his nine players refused to allow guest players and went out, lost 3–0, but played hard and shot constantly until the very end. They never gave up. As he put it, "After the game, they were wasted, but happy and proud of themselves. They knew what they had done." My friend knew that he had taught them at least two things: to love to play, and that doing their best, giving their all, was more important than winning with borrowed players. He was proud of his coaching because he knew that these lessons from sports would carry over into their everyday lives.

If you're getting negative vibes — from your child, other parents, or your own intuition — you must attend games and practices to see for yourself what is going on. Get your information firsthand. When kids don't play well — for lack of experience, or lack of talent — they often complain at home that "It's the coach's fault for not playing me more." Parents naturally want what's best for their kids, so they almost reflexively agree and assume the coach doesn't know what he's doing. It is crucial to appraise the situation objectively yourself before blaming the coach.

If you feel you aren't familiar enough about the sport, talk to other parents. If you're lucky, you'll find some who know what they're talking about and can see more than one side of the picture. Take notes so that you can discuss strengths and weaknesses with either the coach or her supervisor.

Here are some guidelines for examining a coach's strengths and weaknesses, based on the job description above.

Skills Training

- Does the coach demonstrate what he wants (or use a player to demonstrate), or does he just describe it?
- Are practices efficient? Are they fun? Does the coach plan drills so that many kids are active at the same time, or do most of them stand around watching others work? (Standing around is boring for the kids and disrespectful of their time.) Do the drills incorporate technical skills, fitness, and tactics simultaneously, or do they address only one component at a time? Are the kids just passing a ball back and forth (technical), running to a spot and then passing (technical and fitness), or running and passing against a defender (technical, fitness, and tactics)?
- Does the coach tailor practices to fit the needs of the team? (If someone doesn't shoot enough, does he tell her to take thirty shots in fifteen seconds? If the team doesn't pass enough, does he have five players touch the ball before anyone can take a shot? If the team isn't in shape, does he include extra fitness drills in every practice?)
- Is the coach's feedback useful? "You're not hitting well" is negative; the player undoubtedly already knows this, and it doesn't help her improve. What *is* helpful is specific behavioral information to an individual about how to improve her skills, such as "Choke up and use a more open stance," "Remember to square your shoulders to the basket," or "Look up and see where the rest of your teammates are." Players would rather get skill-specific

comments, even if negative ("Don't lunge on defense"), than empty general praise.

- Does the coach encourage players to practice on their own? Does he give them drills to do at home, or a progressive workout routine they can use to get in shape?

Motivating Players

Like parents, coaches have to find a balance between support and pressure to encourage kids to do their best. Concrete, usable feedback helps because it gives direction and guides players in the constant self-evaluation and self-correction that characterize sports.

- Does the coach point out individual progress to each player?
- Does the coach point out the differences between effort and native ability? It's important that the kids know the coach values effort and that while no one has control over results, everyone has control over how hard he works. Eventually, every young athlete understands that working hard increases the odds of achieving the results he wants.
- If the coach plays someone at a position he dislikes or feels doesn't suit his talents, does he explain why? That it's for the good of the team as a whole and he understands that the player is making a sacrifice? That his toughness and sure feet are essential to the defense, where a mistake can mean defeat?
- Does the coach pay attention to each player as a whole person, not just as a talent to be used to win? Does she tell students their first priority is schoolwork and accept a major test or paper as a valid reason to miss a game or practice? (She may excuse this kind of absence once or twice while admonishing the player to plan ahead better and getting tougher if academics consistently interfere.) Does the coach know who responds well to stress and who doesn't? In clutch situations, she must know

whom to call on: not only who is most likely to come through, but also who will suffer most in case of failure — from self-recrimination as well as covert or overt criticism from teammates and parents.

Creating a Team

- Does the coach deploy the available personnel effectively? Does he use different lineups and different strategies against different opponents? (Of course, sports fans argue endlessly about how to deploy resources, so there is not always consensus on what "effective" means in a particular game. The ongoing discussion is one of the passions of participants and spectators alike, and a way to evaluate the intelligence, knowledge, and sophistication of friends and colleagues.)
- Does the coach know who can score or knock opponents down, which players turn over the ball on every possession, who is a reliable pinch hitter, who makes usable passes, who may not be able to score but can block shots and get rebounds? This point relates to disagreements about sound deployment. Parents and players often feel that the coach has evaluated the players' skill incorrectly. Bear in mind, however, that the coach may agree with the families about the players' abilities but have a different philosophy of the game.
- In sum, does he know all the aspects of the game (not just who scores)?

Creating a team requires not just knowledge of the play but also of social dynamics.

- Does the coach develop a sense of belonging, camaraderie, and commitment among the players? Does he encourage group activities, such as team dinners? Being part of a team — being a contributing, respected member of a community with a common goal — is one of the joys of sports. Does he help the players understand that membership on a team is a two-way interaction, between coach and player as well as between player and player? It entails player responsibilities — such as coming to practices and games ready to work, which may mean skipping a late-night party the night before a game.

- When players skip games or practices, does the coach find out why the player didn't show up? Is it a one-time emergency or an ongoing pattern? Whether or not to sanction a player depends to some extent on the goals of the team. Is the purpose to have fun and have everyone play? Is it to teach and improve skills? Is it a competitive team whose purpose is to win? (These goals should be explicit and clear to all members, including the parents, when the player signs up for the team.)

- Whatever the goal, is the coach consistent in what he says and how he deals with issues? If the league requires him to play an automatic rotation, he should play everyone, in that order, and not change it against a particularly strong team. If he says he will bench players who miss practice, he should not change his policy when strong players are the absentees. He can also say that playing time will be dependent on productivity and that life is unfair in the way it distributes talent. Whatever he says, does he follow through on his message with appropriate action?

- How does the coach develop the bench? All seniors eventually graduate, and next year he'll need the players he might currently ignore. Does he include all players in his huddles (not just the starters) so that they can become familiar with his plays, strategies, and thinking patterns? Does he make all players feel they belong and are respected?

- Does the coach listen well — to the players, the parents, the officials? His decisions are his own, but decisions based on more information are usually better than those based on less information.

A Lose–Lose Situation

A high school football coach was adamant that all his players attend August preseason training. One year, a junior, a talented player with great athletic intelligence, missed preseason because he was traveling overseas with his family. The coach, angered by what he considered his weak commitment, retaliated by not playing the boy all fall. His rigidity was lose–lose for everyone. The team lost the talents of this player; the coach looked petty in the eyes of his team; the player felt humiliated and failed to improve his skills. The following year, when the coach really needed him, this player did not come out for football but opted for soccer instead. A lesser penalty would have been sufficient — for example, benching the player until a period equivalent to preseason had elapsed (but insisting, of course, that he attend every practice), or sending him down to JV for a couple of weeks — to have him compete and stay fit, while ensuring that his "transgression" had consequences.

Teaching Respect

Besides teaching respect for one's teammates (arriving on time, ready to work, at all practices and games), coaches should also teach respect for the game and for oneself. Respect for the game means playing by the rules and exhibiting sportsmanship. As one high school coach says, he wants his teams to learn "to win with class and to lose with class."

- Does the coach ignore offensive language, cheating, and fighting, or excuse it ("The opponents were getting really physical")? Or does he take control and reprimand the offender verbally or sanction him (bench him, not start him, suspend him from the team for one or two games, or, if necessary, kick him off the team)?

- Does the coach help his players distinguish between aggression (physical behavior with intent to win) and hostility (excessive roughness, or physical behavior with intent to injure)? Trying to injure another player is simply unacceptable. It violates the whole point of sports — which is to do one's best within a controlled environment of rules. There can be no pride in winning a game by breaking the rules or causing harm to others. If parents find that a coach is encouraging his players to injure an opponent or start a fight ("Take him out! Go for his knees!"), they should act immediately. Get on the cell phone and call the cops if necessary — and it is necessary in the case of assault. They can also work to get another coach. Not only is it wrong ethically, wrong for the long-term character development of the players, but instigating injury to opponents is also beginning to have legal consequences: lawsuits are being brought against organizations and individuals who are in a position to prevent such assaults.
- How does the coach deal with poor officiating? She needs to stand up for her team so they're not penalized by mistakes in officiating, but she shouldn't be abusive. It is not useful to scream "Hey, hometown ref!" or "Whattaya, blind, ump?," which not only sets a bad example but is unlikely to achieve what she wants: fairer calls for her team. A more constructive approach is to call out "Traveling!" or "Palming!" and hope the ref calls the violations or fouls, or at least gives her team a makeup call. (Some officials will penalize coaches for this sort of behavior, but if the coach desists when warned, the players will learn from the example of her effort and her quick response to new information.) The most effective route is to ask the ref quietly to watch for specific infractions that she thinks are going uncalled ("Please watch red number ten for elbows").
- How does the coach behave after a loss? Does he throw a tantrum, screaming at his players or the opponents, at the officials? Does he blame individual players and describe each bad

play in detail to make sure the team knows who he thinks was at fault? Or does he tell the players what they did well and what their opponents did better, that they worked hard and will do better next time?

Here's what I heard one girls' lacrosse coach say at halftime: "We got a foul for not wearing goggles properly. I don't want to know who it was, don't even tell me, but this shouldn't happen again, because we are in complete control of the goggles." This coach successfully reminded her team about the rules for specific equipment, taught them about proper attitude ("we are in control"), and made her point without blaming any one player.

Meeting with Parents

It is almost always helpful for the coach to hold a meeting for parents to discuss the team's objectives, what the coach considers success, how he allocates time, what he expects of his players. Even if the parents' views are not in alignment with the coach's, they will know ahead of time what he is working for.

At such a parents' meeting, the coach should probably also:

- Go over the rules of the game.
- Discuss what's a foul and what isn't in ambiguous situations (how high is high-sticking in field hockey, the difference between a legal screen and an illegal pick, why an obvious foul in soccer might not be called if the offensive team has a tactical advantage).
- Help parents learn how to watch the game: the patterns of offense and defense, who's consistently making assists, who's turning over the ball, who's getting past their defender, who's winning fifty–fifty balls, who's consistently hitting the cut-off man.

Parents who have not grown up watching sports — for example, many mothers — and even parents who have two kids who have played the same sport seriously for years find this kind of review surprisingly helpful. It reminds everyone that the skills are difficult to master, the play of the game is complicated, the rules are also complicated, and that it's better to know what one is talking about before screaming at the coach or the ref.

Dealing with Playing Time

Playing time is usually the most contentious issue between coach and player. First off, playing is the reason to be on the team. It's fun, and it's a chance to show your stuff to peers and adults and earn attention and respect. Second, it's a visible measure of the coach's assessment of a player's talent and effort. Minutes begin to become a major issue beginning around age seven. No one ever thinks he gets enough playing time unless he plays the entire game. Even if a player asks to be subbed out because he's gasping for breath, he usually thinks the coach doesn't get him back in the game quickly enough. This is one of the facts of athletic life. And the issue is not merely the number of minutes, but *which* minutes. Most athletes dream of being the last-ditch, go-to player when the team is behind and needs to score — the one to take the shot at the buzzer or to step up to bat in the bottom of the ninth, the visible and acknowledged savior of the team. They want to be on the field at the end of the game — unless it has already been clearly won or lost, in which case they understand it's time for the bench to come in.

The desire for playing time is complicated by the athlete's desire to win. Unless your child is one of the team's dominant players, these two goals conflict, an unhappy position for most children — as well as for the coach and parents. Many children complain to their parents that the coach doesn't know what he's doing. "I go to every practice and work really hard; it's not fair, I'm as good as the kids who get more time."

Again, it's important to attend games to see what's going on. Maybe the coach *is* favoring certain players, in which case you can survey other parents and speak to her about her lineups. But maybe the kids getting more minutes are in fact more talented than yours, as difficult as that is to admit to yourself or your child. It's also possible that your child is simply complaining to get your sympathy and to finagle more attention or "stuff" from you.

Young kids tend to believe in absolutes (black and white is easier than nuance), and for them one basic absolute rule is that good things are to be divided equally, no matter what. Fortunately, most young kids play on teams set up for fun and learning, so there is little conflict between their beliefs and the need to win. By fifth or sixth grade, if not earlier, kids start becoming aware of who is superior in various activities and where they themselves rank in the hierarchy of talent. This is also the stage in development when winning becomes important. Usually, kids are willing to accept the coach's allocating more time to the impact players, but they also resent playing fewer minutes than players whom they judge to be at or close to their own level.

Kids also need to come to terms with the sad fact that, indeed, life is unfair. Talent is distributed unequally at birth. Some kids seem to be born with the ability to throw a ball 70 mph, or dribble — with either feet or hands — ambidextrously. Sometimes sports — and coaches — can help kids become reconciled to this fact. Another unequally distributed talent is the aptitude for working hard. Sometimes sports — and coaches — can help develop this aptitude, which will stand the player in good stead throughout life.

Do your best to be objective in judging your child's abilities. Pretend he's someone else's kid and see how he measures up. Or ask a knowledgeable friend to watch a game and give his candid opinion. (This can be risky, however. Many parents can bear anything but criticism of their children; you must be prepared to listen to a negative evaluation without being offended or holding it against your friend. If you don't think you can manage that, it's not worth risking a friendship.) Once you've seen for yourself, you will be better able to help your child deal with the playing-time issue.

If your child is young, consider enrolling him in a recreational league that stipulates a minimum amount of playing time (three-quarters of the game, or automatic rotations of the lineup) for each player. Even in these leagues, however, discretionary playing time is often allocated by ability.

If your child is older, suggest that she ask the coach what he's looking for in his players, what she can do to improve her game and get more time. Once she knows what he considers her weaknesses to be, she can work on these areas in practice. Regarding practice, you can also point out to your child that athletes practice to get better, not to get minutes.

✳

As I discussed in Chapter 2, parents are elated when their child is successful. One essential characteristic of athletics is that success is measurable, visible, and publicly acknowledged. Many kids are excellent at running fast, making baskets, scoring touchdowns, catching a fly ball. And their prowess is reflected in the score.

As kids grow older and become more sophisticated players, however, excellence can be more difficult to ascertain. While scoring is exciting and the objective of the game, scores are often made possible only by an essential but less evident block by a lineman, or by another player's cutting to the basket and drawing defenders. And sometimes a prominent, flashy player — perhaps a boy who is brilliant at threading his way through defenders to bring the ball up the sidelines — wastes his efforts by consistently taking unmakable shots. He looks great but is not productive.

Assessing performance accurately is harder than it looks once players understand the game. It helps if you've played the sport, but even if you're a novice, you can learn by watching attentively as often as possible. Over time, you'll become more knowledgeable about the skills and tactics involved as well as the ongoing contributions of individual players.

Before urging the coach to give your child more minutes, consider the possible reasons for his decisions and be sure to take into account the nuances of strategy and execution.

My child gets hardly any time on his middle school basketball team. He knows he's not as good as most of the other boys — they've all been playing for years. I think the school should be teaching him how to improve and should play everyone on the team.

There are several issues here. Should the school be teaching your child how to play basketball better? Yes. Is he improving? Does he think so? Do you?

What is the school's philosophy of middle school teams? Is it inclusion: everyone gets approximately equal amounts of time? A compromise between inclusion and winning: everyone plays a minimum amount of time (maybe a third of a game) but the superior players get more time? Or is it preparation and winning: middle school teams train players for junior varsity and thus use lineups constructed to win? Seventh and eighth grade is about when kids begin to think that winning is important, so any of these philosophies is appropriate.

A parallel situation to consider is that solos in school orchestra concerts are assigned to kids who are superior musicians, and they're usually the ones who take private instrumental lessons. Is this unfair? If you think yes, what other criteria should be applied?

If your child is committed to basketball, you can sign him up to play on an outside team. Ask the coaches in the athletic department about local leagues. You can also suggest that he practice on his own in your driveway, or practice left- and right-handed dribbling in the living room. If he's not that interested, you might have him consider another sport or an entirely different activity, such as writing for the school newspaper or trying out for the school play.

Suggesting Changes

The kids on my son's hockey team complain they're not fit — they run out of gas in the third period. What's the best way to suggest more fitness drills to the coach?

Speaking to the coach is like speaking to a teacher. Do your homework (observe and gather evidence), be respectful, and offer concrete, constructive suggestions. When meeting with the coach, you or your son should describe the situation as clearly as you can, assume the coach has reasons for what he's doing (this is very different from assuming the coach is a jerk), and find out what the reasons are. Then you or he might suggest alternative ways of handling practice.

In addition, when your son complains about these issues, ask him, "What are you going to do about it?" If players are aware they aren't fit, they can go to the weight room or the track on their own, either individually or as a team. It's more fun to work out together but harder to organize. Even if the coach is in fact a jerk, the kids need to take some responsibility for their own training and effort. They know what they want — fitness — and they know how to achieve it. They can also ask the athletic trainer to help them set up a fitness regimen. They shouldn't depend on someone else, especially a coach they don't respect, to get them to do the right thing.

My daughter's school basketball coach is incompetent. The players haven't learned anything over the season (they're still making bad passes, but now scoring fewer free throws, doing less on defense), and he calls time-outs on his own team's fast breaks. The team routinely loses by thirty points a game. My daughter loves basketball. Is there anything I can do?

Talk to the other team parents and see whether they concur that the primary weakness of the team is the coach. If so, you might write a group letter to the school's athletic director detailing your concerns. It would also be helpful to have the players write their own letter, signed by as many players as possible.

Be as specific as you can about your complaints, and provide evidence when possible. Try to be balanced in your appraisal: Include the coach's strengths as well. Give credence to other causes for the team's poor showing. Are the other teams in the league exceptionally strong this year? Is the team lacking in talent or height this year? Has it been plagued by more injuries than usual? A one-sided rant is not usually persuasive. Besides, the A.D. hired this coach; he must think the guy has something going for him.

If possible, compare the credentials and experience of your school's coach with those of the other coaches in the league. Include suggestions about how the coach can get extra training (such as coaching clinics) or where the A.D. can look for a replacement.

After delivering your letter, ask for a meeting with the A.D. and a small group of parents (a large group is intimidating, hard to manage, and usually produces unfocused, uninformative discussion). Choose the attendees carefully: you want parents who agree that the coach is inadequate; who are reasonable, articulate, know what they're talking about; and who have children who are starters and therefore have some clout with the department.

My son's soccer coach plays favorites. He says if a kid misses practice he won't start him. But the most skilled player on the team often misses practice and the coach starts him anyway. The kid is good but not that good, plus he doesn't always give 100 percent.

Before talking to the coach, figure out what you want and why you want things changed. Is your son complaining about the inconsistent application of stated policy? Do you think your child deserves more time or starts than he's getting? Do you wish he played a different position? Do you wish he were more talented than he actually is? What does your son want from the team?

If, after careful, calm analysis, you and your son believe that the coach's inconsistency is detrimental to the team as a whole, the two of you, or you alone, might talk to the coach in private about the importance of consistency of message and behavior. The coach should mean what he says and act on it.

It's easy and clear to say minutes or starting depends on attendance; it's difficult and messy to say they depend on productivity. Find out whether the coach uses attendance as the criterion because it's convenient, quantifiable, and easy to explain, or because he believes in rewarding the act of showing up. At a certain age, however, effort alone is not enough; results are important too (and not just in sports).

Evaluating productivity demands knowledge, observation, and judgment, and even experts disagree on the worth of different players. (Who was a better quarterback — Johnny Unitas or Joe Montana? Who was the best big man — Wilt, Kareem, or Bill [Walton or Russell]? And don't forget George Mikan.) How good is this skilled guy on the team? Can he do things no one else on the team can? Trap any ball and have the vision and skill to redirect it to the only open player? Dribble through three defenders and shoot into an upper corner of the goal? If he can do these things without attending every practice or giving 100 percent, he deserves the minutes — and the coach should stop saying that he'll bench kids who don't show up for practice.

Of course it's not fair that some kids are born with star talent and give little in return, but in the cosmic scheme of things, that's the way it is. One great benefit of sports is helping kids learn to deal with this phenomenon constructively — by practicing harder or coming to a philosophical equilibrium that accepts the unfairness of outcomes while embracing the satisfaction of making the effort or fighting the good fight.

Coaching Boys, Coaching Girls

Coaches say, "Teach the boys to pass and teach the girls to shoot." (A parallel saying for older competitors is: "Male lawyers need sensitivity training and women lawyers need insensitivity training.") Anson Dorrance, legendary coach of the University of North Carolina women's soccer team, says, "Men respond to your strength, women respond to your humanity." He says what's important to women is connection: "Women are more sensitive and more demanding of each other. . . . Men are not sensitive and not demanding of each other, and that's a wonderful combination for building team chemistry." Whether the differences are biological or socially constructed, and whether or not these differences recede as Title IX gains more ground, most people agree that that's the way it is.

Parents of girls need to be aware of these differences in order to evaluate the effectiveness of their daughters' coaches, and in the case of complaints, to determine whether the cause is lack of sports knowledge or a mismatch in communications style.

One long-time college soccer coach recounts how the culture of girls' sports has changed over the past ten years. He started off with a girls' club team at an Ivy League school. If it rained at practice, when he turned around to sub in his bench players he'd find that they had simply gone back to the dorm to get out of the wet. The other thing that drove him crazy was that if a player knocked an opponent over, she would stop, apologize profusely, and help the opponent up. Over the years, and after much yelling on his part, the girls stopped apologizing but still extended a helping hand. Now, he's relieved to see, the girls routinely knock their opponents over as part of the game.

Girls Are More Social

During halftime at soccer or basketball games, boys of all ages run into the empty space and start kicking or shooting the ball. Girls huddle around the sidelines and chat.

As a broad generalization, boys are interested in achievement, girls are interested in social relationships. Boys just want to play. They crave the game, the physical contact, the win–lose status, the demonstration of their own and their teammates' proficiency. They are not particularly concerned with who's on their team as long as they're good. Girls are more interested in the process. Girls want to have good players on their team, but they also want to like their teammates. They judge players not only by their skill level and productivity, but also by how nice they are, how trustworthy, and whether they're friends, or potential friends. It's important to girls to enjoy spending time with their teammates. If they don't like someone, they often won't pass to her. As one coach put it, "I have to tell the girls to be respectful toward each to reach the common goal. I don't need to have this conversation with boys." They already know the point is to play and preferably to win.

Parents who have both sons and daughters frequently remark on the dramatic differences in the warm-up period before a game. Boys arrive, put on their equipment, and warm up. Girls wave greetings to each new arrival when she's thirty yards away, hug and kiss each other, and chat as they dress. More than one coach, after suffering enormous frustration at how much longer girls take to prepare than boys, has resigned himself to reality and told girls to arrive forty-five minutes before game time instead of the thirty minutes that boys need. Thus they build in a period for socializing but still have enough time to warm up.

Girls are less reductive than boys. Even dedicated female athletes tend to see a larger picture of themselves and their circle, beyond the athletic field: they're friends, they're photographers or musicians, they're good students and school leaders. Boys, on the other hand, when they're on the field, and perhaps when off the field as well, tend to confine their identity to the athletic prowess of themselves and their teammates.

Girls are more aware of themselves as part of a larger whole, their team, but also of their role as a whole person with many attributes. They tend to be "team players," willing to pass to the open man (unless they despise her), whereas boys are more aware of their own stats and are more apt to make a play that makes them shine as an individual. Most girls will help a fallen opponent up when the play is over. Many older boys' teams start fights with their opponents. This is not an isolated phenomenon; I have noticed these differences on every level of athletic team I have worked with, from grade school kids through college.

Different Ways with Language

Boys and girls treat each other's weaknesses differently. Boys tease, girls console. As a college basketball coach points out: "If a guy goes coast to coast and blows the layup, he's going to hear about it for a long time, from everyone — from the starters, from the bench, from the coach. Unless it's the play that loses the game, in which case no one says anything. On the other hand, if a girl goes coast to coast and blows the layup, her teammates say things like, 'It's okay, don't worry about it, you'll get it next time.'"

One long-standing tradition of sports is jock humor, or the reverse insult. A coach, for example, might taunt a team star who conspicuously misses an easy goal by calling him "blind boy" for the rest of the afternoon, or call a girl "the turnover queen" after a bad day on the basketball court. Boys generally understand this as an inverted compliment, because most coaches would not subject a less able player to this type of razzing. Girls, however, unaccustomed to this form of discourse, hear only the insult and not the intention, and they can become enraged. (This is bad for both coach and player, because rage usually decreases productivity.)

While it is a good idea for coaches (and parents) to learn to talk to girls differently from boys on the athletic field (especially since Title IX has brought so many girls into athletics), it is also a good idea for girls to learn that caustic badinage is how many people talk in the real world, particularly the work world. Girls need to learn to deal with this, either by changing the model by presenting an alternative way of talking, for example, or by using rough teasing themselves. At the very least they must learn to get over feeling hurt by any verbal insult.

Coaches of girls should also be aware that girls are extremely sensitive about their appearance and weight, much more so than boys are. This concern of girls' is compounded in those sports where weight makes a significant difference, such as gymnastics, skating, and dancing. Coaches should be wary of mentioning weight gratuitously; if they're concerned about fitness, they can discuss this with the girls in terms of outcomes rather than weight. Don't say, "You're out of shape; you need to drop at least five pounds." Do say, "You're not as fit as you could be; let's start a running program to increase your stamina."

Reacting to Criticism and Praise

Girls take criticism more personally than boys do. The branch of psychology known as attribution theory finds that females tend to attribute their failures to their own inherent shortcomings (lack of effort or skill), whereas males tend to assume an external cause of failure (the talent of the opposition, bad timing). Girls often hear criticism of their playing as criticism of themselves as a whole being. Thus if a soccer coach says, "You're striking the ball wrong," a girl tends to respond, "I'm lousy, aren't I?"

Coach: No, I mean you're striking it with the wrong part of your foot.

Girl: I knew it — I'm really no good.

Coach: No, just do it differently.

A boy, in contrast, hears the coach say, "You're striking the ball wrong" and understands that he's to change the way he kicks the ball.

Because girls tend to define themselves in terms of a social network, they are more prickly about being criticized in front of their peers than boys are. Coaches find it more effective to take them aside to talk to them. It's also easier for girls to listen to negative comments when they're balanced by positive observations. ("You were great on rebounding today, but your passes were too hard. Think about how to make passes that the receiver can use.") Boys are more accustomed to blunt criticism, and some boys don't hear what a coach says *unless* the remarks are blunt.

Girls and boys respond to challenges differently as well. If during a boys' game a coach screams to a player, "You're not hustling!," often that player's response is "I'll show you!," and he knocks himself out to prove the coach wrong. When the same coach screams the same words to a girl, he's more likely to see the girl sag her shoulders and give up.

Another difference is how boys and girls hear a coach's praise of their teammates. Some very observant coaches point out that when a coach compliments a male athlete — "Jack had a great game, played great on defense today" — his teammates hear this as a positive reward for Jack and think, "Yeah, he played great today." But with girls, when a coach says, "Jill had a great game, played great on defense today," her teammates think, "Well, what about me? I played hard today and I got a lot of rebounds. Why isn't Coach talking about me too?" What coaches find effective with girls is to spread the praise around. "If you tend to praise one too much or too often, the other females react and get sullen or annoyed," one coach notes.

Statements of intent are also heard differently. If a coach says, "You did great today at practice; I'm starting you tomorrow," girls hear that as a promise. If the coach changes his mind, they take it personally as a broken promise and hold this against him as a character defect. Boys seem to accept changes of mind more easily because they hear statements of intent as casual utterances of the moment.

Why is this? Who knows? (Cue Henry Higgins: "Why can't a woman be more like a man?")

Male Coaches, Female Players

Male coaches of females are subject to a double standard. A female coach can talk to both male and female players about their social life, drugs, alcohol. She can baby-sit young players and invite teams to a sleepover at her home. A male coach can't do the same things without people raising at least an eyebrow, if not a stink.

Some parents are concerned about any physical contact between male coaches and female players. The essence of sports is physicality, and most sports involve physical contact of some sort. In general, female athletes say that having a male coach put his arm on their shoulder indicates acceptance and is not at all predatory or intimidating. The male coach does the same thing, they point out, to male athletes. Patting a player on the buttocks, however, is a different matter and should be avoided. *Note*: While the stereotype is of male coaches harassing female players, harassment also takes place male to male, female to female, and female to male.

In very rare instances, coaches, male or female, will abuse the power of their authority and touch or harass players inappropriately. Players should be aware that they have the right to say "That makes me uncomfortable." Players should also keep records of any incidents they find troubling, and talk to their teammates and friends about the situation. Some schools tell coaches not to spend time alone with any player — to avoid driving an individual kid home or training one-on-one, or taking one student to a professional game or tournament. Small groups of kids make the situation more comfortable for everyone. Getting permission from the parents for any of these special occasions is always a good idea.

Parents need to observe the relationship between the individual coach and individual player to decide what's acceptable or not. It is unfair to suspect that a particular coach will act inappropriately simply because other coaches have harassed or abused players. Everything depends on the individuals involved and their repeated patterns of behavior.

Most adult–pupil relationships are positive and productive. In a few rare instances, they become exploitative, and when such abuses become known, they receive tremendous amounts of public attention. If you have concerns, based on actual and repeated behavior, discuss them with your child and the adult as early as possible.

The Box Score

- The coach must be able to teach.
- Do your homework before judging the coach (know the sport and attend the games).
- Be as objective as possible about your child's performance.
- Be respectful and constructive when seeking to change the coach's methods and behavior.
- The goal is for the players to improve their skills, work hard in games, develop good values, and learn to love and respect their sport.

Chapter 4

To Every Thing
There Is a Season

INSTILLING A SENSE OF PERSPECTIVE

*Keeping sports from taking over your life can be difficult,
but it is possible by keeping your values in mind and taking
the long-term view.*

An Ohio father described the coach of his daughter's middle school basketball team as a yeller: He screams at the girls for every mistake. In one game, the score was 60–2 in his favor (the father was praying for the other team to reach 10), and the coach was screaming because the girls let in the 2 points. After the game, instead of being elated, three girls on the winning team were weeping, and the father suggested to the coach that yelling at the players was unnecessary, since they had won. The other parents, including those whose daughters were crying, reprimanded this father for making the coach "feel bad."

A fourth-grade basketball team in California reached the finals of their town league. The parent-volunteer coach wanted his team to have extra practice, but the only time he could get a full court was 2:00 p.m. the day before the game, when the kids were still in school. He told his players to get early-dismissal notes from their parents with fake excuses like dentist appointments so they could attend practice. The kids' school, puzzled when two parents called asking why they were being asked to lie, investigated and discovered that nine other parents had gone along with the ruse. Furthermore, the parent coach could not comprehend why anyone thought his plan was a bad idea. (The next year he transferred his son to a private school.)

Both these stories illustrate a failure, on several fronts, to keep sports in balance with other aspects of life. Win-at-all-costs is a losing attitude; so is sports-at-all-costs. In a culture that is sports-mad, paying professional athletes vastly more than virtually anyone else, where kids pursue athletics to gain attention, respect, and scholarships, it's often difficult to remember that there is anything more important than playing and winning. But in fact, millions of people live fulfilling, productive lives without ever throwing or kicking a ball.

Lack of perspective on sports often results in undesirable outcomes: family life can cease to exist, athletes can experience overwhelming stress, athletes can come to think that winning is the only thing or that the everyday rules don't apply to them.

When a family's life revolves around sports and getting their kids to practices and games for various teams three seasons a year, or even all year round, many parents ask if their children are doing too much. Unfortunately, there's seldom an easy answer.

How Much Is Too Much?

Sports participation is great for kids, but there *is* such a thing as too much. If the student can no longer balance the activities in her life, if she can't keep up with her schoolwork, hang with friends, daydream, read a book for fun once in a while, do some community service, attend religious services, do her share of the family chores, *and* get to her practices and games, then perhaps she needs to cut back on sports. Not that she can do all of these things as much as she would like (hardly anyone can) — being on a competitive team sometimes means not seeing friends, not going to the movies all season. But can she do most of them? Does she feel like she's sacrificing too much to be on a team? Is her schoolwork suffering?

Teenagers routinely live with a great deal of stress and seldom welcome unsolicited suggestions from their parents. Athletes who play on travel teams or at even higher levels, going beyond neighboring towns for games and tournaments, live with more stress than most. The long hours spent practicing and traveling to and participating in competitions strain them physically, but also socially and academically.

Some parents think that putting their athletic sons on multiple teams keeps them busy and out of trouble. Sometimes the players thrive, but I also see cases where the kids turn surly because they're under so much pressure. I've seen some who play on three teams in one season, and that easily leads to burnout. Besides the emotional toll, burning out is especially troubling because one of the great benefits of sports is encouraging the habit of lifelong physical activity, and some kids who burn out are "turned off" sports for many years, sometimes forever.

I also hear about parents who drag their kids out of bed every Saturday morning to go to the batting cages for extra practice, or who force their kids to shoot a hundred foul shots every night in the backyard or driveway. They think they're doing their kids a favor by instilling discipline and improving their skills, but usually the result is kids who drop out and never return.

The point when sports participation becomes "too much," however, is completely individual, differing for every athlete, whether child or teen. Let the athlete, whatever age, help decide with you, rather than your deciding for her. Two kids might start for the same middle school soccer team, but one might be having the time of her life, enjoying the camaraderie, the competition, the experience, while the other can't wait for practice to end. The issues might be mental — "I don't enjoy competing against other people" — or physical — "My body hurts when I run a lot in soccer practice" or "I'm scared of getting hurt because the opponents are so much bigger than I am." Parents must be receptive to these concerns and try to figure out why their children are not having fun. It's important not to force kids or teens into playing: it won't be fun for them or for you.

The decision about how much sports participation is right for a specific child must be made by his or her family. If the athlete is stressed out or irritable, developing headaches or stomachaches, think about cutting back on sports. If kids are having fun, and if their grades aren't suffering and they aren't getting hurt, let them play. Sports sure beat a lot of other things that kids and teens can do with their free time!

But it isn't just the young athlete whose needs must be considered. Often, the whole family sacrifices when a child plays on a high-level team. Family dinners, or just plain time together as a family, become rare. Parents may lavish time, attention, and emotional focus on the star athlete, and can skimp on the less visible needs of other family members. Financial resources flow toward equipment, fees, trainers, tutors, transportation and hotel costs. It's hard on the family and often very hard on the other children, who feel neglected.

When the family as a whole seems to be suffering, it's up to the parents to step back and consider what to do. What are the long-range goals for each child? What are the benefits and costs of working toward each child's long-range goals? The parents must examine the allocation of the family resources — financial, emotional, logistical — and make sure that no child is being shortchanged.

If the star athlete is consuming an unfair share of these resources, point this out to him and ask him for suggestions on how he can restore some balance. For example, he can arrange rides with other families; he can get a summer job and contribute some of his earnings to help pay for his equipment or tournament expenses; he can attend his siblings' games (or piano recitals or debating matches) and help coach their performance.

Warning Signs of Too Much Sports

The athlete

- Is tense, moody, and irritable almost all the time, especially around practice and game times.
- Is doing badly academically.
- Pursues almost no other activities besides sports (no painting, singing, journalism).
- Has little time to relax or see friends.
- Is primarily focused on improving his athletic skills and has little time for participating in or serving the community around him.
- Treats games as an obligation rather than fun.
- Is reluctant to go to games or practice.
- Is exhausted during the school day.

Most high school and college athletes think of these years of playing for their school as a wonderful time in their lives. They're having fun and improving their skills, most are doing well academically, and they're gaining recognition and admiration from their friends as well as from strangers. Sometimes, however, the stresses of athletics are overwhelming.

If you see in your child more than four or more of the warning signs listed above, talk to her about cutting back on her sports schedule. Ask her to think about what she's giving up and whether it's worth it.

Balancing Athletics and Academics

Students, especially in middle and high school, should be students first and athletes second. What they need to see them through life is a mastery of basic skills and enough familiarity with natural and historical phenomena to confirm or question other people's arguments about how the world works. If you let your children take easy courses for the sake of maintaining athletic eligibility, your short-sightedness shortchanges them. They miss out on learning challenging content as well as discovering how to study; they also learn that the grownups around them consider athletics more important than anything else.

Help your athlete manage both his schoolwork and his athletic activity. Time management is the key.

Time Management

Some time management tips to suggest to your child:

- Plan ahead. Make prioritized to-do lists every day (show him your own to-do lists). For things due tomorrow, start with the most complicated, difficult items while you're still fresh. Use a kitchen timer to signal when you need to be somewhere else.
- Start major projects early. Remember that everything takes longer than you think it will (and if a project takes less time, you have a bonus in extra time).
- Break tasks down into smaller units — it makes them less overwhelming.
- Use your energies efficiently. When is your peak period? Morning? Afternoon? Evening? Plan your work schedule accordingly.
- Take breaks but use the time well: avoid watching television or playing Free Cell; pick up your room or empty the dishwasher instead. Even switching from your English paper to your math problems can refresh your brain cells.
- Nap when you need to or when you can — even short naps (ten to fifteen minutes) help — and get to bed early so you get enough sleep at night.
- Keep long-term goals in mind so you don't waste time. Cut out television altogether during the sports season. Don't answer the phone (it disrupts concentration); get an answering machine.

Elite Athletes

One mother complained that her daughter, a state-level gymnast, was constantly crabby and stressed out. The girl worried about her rankings, about her academic performance, about the fact that she never saw her friends. The other gymnasts she knew were extremely competitive, as were their families.

This is a tough situation. I suggested that in a calm moment, this mother ask her daughter whether she recognizes what she is paying to stay in a highly competitive individual sport. Spending hours in the gym every day, competing in the state championships, and working to get to the nationals make for a grueling schedule. These goals are hard on the body, and they make getting homework done extremely difficult. Ask her whether this is how she wants to spend her high school years. She has a choice to make, and she is responsible for that choice. No one is forcing her to do gymnastics.

The family can establish conditions that the athlete must meet if she is to continue.

- She cannot be rude to others, particularly her parents.
- She must express appreciation to the family for their support, for getting her to and from the gym and tournaments.
- She must maintain a specified grade point average.

If she fails to meet these standards, she must quit. (If you set up conditions, you must impose the consequences if she fails. Otherwise you will be teaching her that you don't mean what you say and that her athletic performance is so important to *you* that you will allow her to shortchange her education and act like a spoiled brat — the rules of normal behavior don't apply to her.)

You can also try to reduce her level of stress by pointing out, again in a calm moment, that she can only be responsible for what she can control. She is in control of her attitude, her effort, and her preparation in her sport. She is not responsible for the outcome, that is, the judges' score.

Also be sure that she knows, from your words and your behavior, that you love her no matter how she does in her sport.

Are Sports Worth the Sacrifice?

If you think your child is overly focused on sports, have him picture himself in the future, looking back at his high school athletic career. Have him consider these two questions for balance:

1. *Was it worth it?* The injuries, the stress, the missed family dinners, the time not spent with friends? Could his grades have been better if he hadn't spent so much time on sports? Could he have done more community service? Could he have explored other areas of interest, or even other sports?
2. *Did he give it his best shot?* Was there anything else he could have done to improve his athletic performance? Did he train as hard as he could? Study the game and his opponents to gain the best advantage?

The crabby gymnast decided she wanted to compete at a Division I college. She loved her sport and knew she would always regret not attempting to fulfill this ambition, even if she failed to make such a team. She transferred from her academically demanding high school, which was far away from the gym, to one geared toward young professionals and kids with a passion they need to pursue. She is much happier with a less competitive academic workload and feels freer during her hours at the gym. She believes that her sense of commitment and dedication to her sport is an important part of who she is, and she is certain she has made the right decision for herself.

A patient of mine is a nationally ranked runner who loves running but is also a talented basketball player and actress. She will continue running, but she will not give up basketball or theater, which she describes as cooperative, collaborative endeavors that make her feel fully alive. Many coaches encourage her to focus exclusively on track, but she says she's not Olympic material, and besides, that isn't who she is. She would be unhappy if she gave up her other interests.

Group (Mis)Behavior: "Jocks Rule"

Psychologists have established that people in groups can be incited to do things they would not do on their own. Being part of a group seems to muffle personal inhibitions as well as a sense of personal responsibility ("If everyone's doing it, I can't be blamed") — a volatile and unhappy combination. Given that adolescents have an intense need to be part of a group, parents must be on the alert for group situations that lead to risk-taking and delinquent behavior.

As a special sphere separate from everyday life, sports can give athletes, coaches, and fans a sense of belonging to a special group, a sense that exempts them from the ordinary rules of behavior. Most of us are all too familiar with the lurid stories: the player who tries to strangle his coach, the coach who tries to strangle his player, the player who spits at the umpire, and worse. In Glen Ridge, New Jersey, some high school football players sexually assaulted a retarded girl; several Texas high school state champion football players are serving sentences of ten to twenty-six years for armed robbery.

Players, fans, league officials, and sports commentators may call such behavior extreme and unacceptable, but those in charge frequently fail to take action. So driven are some adults to be affiliated with a winning team or player that they overlook misbehavior (drunkenness, drunk driving, vandalism, petty theft) on the grounds that "boys will be boys" and the team needs the guilty players in order to win. Some even claim that offenders need the support of the team to straighten out. If the surrounding community of adults think that athletes deserve special treatment, the athletes will learn that the rules don't apply to them. Further, since most teenagers are impelled to test limits, they keep upping the ante of misbehavior to see what they can get away with.

To raise athletes well, the adults in their communities — the parents, coaches, teachers, law enforcement officials — must be sure they all send the same message: Bad behavior is unacceptable. If parents and sheriffs overlook the vandalism or delinquency of athletes, the athletes, and other students, learn that the rules don't apply to the transgressions of athletes. If a coach ignores or snickers at male athletes' pinching girls or calling them insulting names while the school principal condemns this behavior, students become confused and the harassment is almost sure to continue. Because these anti-girl behaviors were condoned for so long, sometimes adults don't know what to say and need to be given a script (e.g., "No name-calling," or "If you touch a girl suggestively, you have to be very sure it's acceptable to her. Otherwise, don't do it").

Teachers, school administrators, law enforcement officials, and coaches need to think about the long-term character development of their student athletes. What do athletes need to learn and do to function as productive people? When should they be cut some slack? A good rule of thumb is to treat athletes the same way that other notable students — the members of the honor society, the winners of the science fair, the stars of the school musical — are treated. Athletes should be given neither more nor fewer privileges than the other standout students.

When male athletes are treated as special, some push to discover the limits of acceptable behavior. They bully nonathletes or younger team members, and harass girls. To some extent, many kids, especially starting in middle school, are mean to each other, perhaps as part of growing up and being insecure about their identity. But adults can help by speaking out and reminding kids that there is no honor in cruelty or bullying, that honor means taking care of those who are weaker than you. Adults can also remind students about the importance of empathy and being fair: "How would you feel if someone did that to you?"

Parents and other adults in the community need to be vigilant and think in terms of the long view for their young athletes. If a team or community is pulling its children into antisocial behavior or attitudes, or worse, it's time to look into changing teams or changing schools.

Parents and the Media

Read the sports pages or watch *SportsCenter* with your kids and point out how the media glorify extreme behavior, which is all too often antisocial and destructive. An athlete may sponsor sports workshops for at-risk students to motivate them to do well in school, but these efforts seldom make the front page, or even the back pages. What does make the front page, and the evening news, is athletes and coaches behaving badly. You know the stories: not just the professional baseball player who spits at the umpire, but the football player who assaults his wife or girlfriend, or arranges to have his pregnant girlfriend shot. And what is featured in the replays? The basketball players who taunt and insult their opponents. The dunk rather than the medium-range jump shot. The baseball bat thrown at another player.

Commentators used to help spectators develop an appreciation of the game itself — the skills of defense, of creating passing lanes, of seizing opportunities that open up suddenly, of making intelligent decisions, of never giving up — but today too many of them are more interested in the feuds, the easy, dramatic one-move score rather than the goal that's developed by several players. It's all contributing to the short attention span of the spectator and trickles down from professional sports through college sports to high school sports.

Help your child understand and deal with the value system reflected and magnified by the media. Ask him why so often the headline sports stories are about bad behavior (to sell papers, to sell advertising time). Ask what is left out, what is needed to construct a more well-rounded story. Talk to him about what you and he admire in an athlete, about the reasons to love and respect the game.

Poor Sportsmanship

The point of playing sports is the joy of moving one's muscles and the satisfaction of mastering skills and tactics in accord with the rules of the game. The mastery is demonstrated in two ways: by comparing your current to past performance, and by comparing your current performance to that of your opponent.

There is no point in not trying to win — games are meant to be won. On the other hand, there's no point in trying to win at all costs — by injuring the opponent or by cheating. The rules give players a standard against which to measure and compare their performance; breaking the rules means there's no standard, no game, and no satisfaction from winning or even doing well.

The essence of sportsmanship is self-control — maintaining tranquillity and perspective in the midst of emotional intensity. Athletics offers an authentic opportunity to develop self-control because it's an activity that kids care deeply about, and one that often leads to extreme behavior.

In high-contact sports, acts that in everyday life would be considered grounds for arrest are considered normal play. When sports like football and hockey encourage, even reward, bone-jarring tackles and ferocious body checks (albeit on players wearing heavy protective padding), articulating the limits of acceptable behavior is difficult. What is the difference between aggression and assault? Some athletes have trouble knowing when to stop being aggressive even after the game ends, and they get into numerous fights.

Sometimes opponents will rough up a player or players systematically, out of sight of the ref. (This is usually an issue only with older kids.) If this happens to your child, remind him that the other team has probably picked him out as an impact player (a compliment), and most important, that getting mad or seeking vengeance will not help his team win. He has to learn to suck it up and keep playing as hard as he can. He can also yell "Stop pushing" or "Let go of me!" In addition, he can approach his coach or captain, who can then politely say to the official, next time he is in earshot, "Could you please keep an eye on blue number ten? He's been pushing our number four." The players should also know they can count on their coach to stand up for them when they feel the officiating is inadequate.

One thing all children must learn is to adjust their play to the ref's whistle. Some officials call stricter games than others, and if the ref allows the game to become very physical, kids should be prepared to play physically rather than complain.

One absolute rule is that players should never deliberately injure another player. Deliberate injury means the player, and possibly the coach or parents, is out of control and has entirely lost sight of the purpose of organized sports.

If a game gets out of hand and turns dangerous, the coach, or a knowledgeable parent, must intervene. If a ref is unable to cool down an extremely physical game, sometimes the only safety measure available to a team is to withdraw from competition.

In a local soccer game, Blue was ahead 5–0, and the Red team, visibly frustrated, began kicking Blue players on the ground, drawing blood (one needed stitches). Amazingly, the ref did not penalize Red. The Blue coach told the ref and the Red coach that if unnecessary roughness continued, her girls would not play. The Red coach said fine, that would be a forfeit. The Blue coach gave her team the choice: continue and win or quit and forfeit. Blue chose to forfeit.

The next day, Blue's athletic director reprimanded the coach for allowing the team to forfeit. The A.D. had succumbed to a short-sighted win-at-all-costs mentality. The parents then met with the principal and the A.D. to discuss the the athletic program and the safety of the students. In addition, the school and parents protested the ref's losing control of the game and made sure he was no longer allowed to officiate in that league.

Coaches and parents should instill habits of good sportsmanship throughout the season, by reminding kids of the difference between aggression and hostility with intent to injure, and by not rewarding bad behavior.

Seemingly small gestures incorporated as a routine part of the game can underscore for athletes and parents the need for respect for the game itself and for others. For example:

- Having the principal or coach welcome the fans before the game and remind them to cheer for their own team and for good moves, but not to insult anyone or be negative to either team, the fans, or the officials.
- Reminding the team (or your child) before the game that the person with the most difficult position on the field is the official. Hardly anyone is ever happy with his performance.
- Reminding players that one bad call seldom changes the outcome of a game. (The missed free throws, turnovers, poor shot decisions, lack of effort are what add up to losing games, and they are not the official's fault.)
- Having the players call the official "Sir" or "Ma'am" and say thank you after the game.
- Shaking hands after the game. This may seem superficial, but some kids take it seriously enough to refuse to do it; some spit on their hands before shaking, or say "Bad game" to their opponents.
- Introducing the official to the players and fans: "This is Stephen Jones. He's the father of two boys who play ice hockey, Max and Peter." Even a description as simple as this often reminds everyone that the official is a human being with a life outside the game.

The coaches and team parents should be alert in general to disrespectful attitudes. When the best soccer player on a team of sixteen-year-old girls was kicked in the ankle by the opponents, she fell and

Be Fair to Officials

As we all know, officials are not perfect. The job is simply beyond human capabilities. (That's why there are so many electronic line demarcations and so much instant replay equipment.) Sometimes officials miss important, game-changing occurrences and need help. This is the justification for teams to celebrate goals as soon as the ball crosses the goal line, and also for indicating physical distress when a foul has occurred — both are signals asking for official intervention that can also be deliberately misused by players.

The official's responsibility is to blow the whistle both ways, that is, call the same fouls on both teams. If an official seems unable to do this, the players must simply play on, not allowing anger to interfere with their performance but letting the coach take care of this on the field. In some leagues, designated observers submit written reports to the league officials.

Before every game, one of my favorite refs tells both teams, "I always do my best not to make mistakes, but I guarantee you I will make mistakes. It's part of the game."

lay on the ground moaning. (She was out for the next two weeks.) The opponents milled around her, laughing and making fun of her within her hearing: "Ooooh, poor baby, she sounds like she's having an orgasm." The adults on the opposing team did nothing to rein in the girls' behavior.

A league can take action to remind parents and players about sportsmanship. For example, a league official can walk around the games and talk to athletes and parents who are becoming over-excited and behaving badly. Some towns, like Jupiter, Florida, and El Paso, Texas, are requiring parents to take a sportsmanship workshop in order to register their children in the town athletic leagues. Some leagues have instituted "Silent Weekends," when parents are to say nothing, not even cheer, during the games. The Coast Soccer Premier League of Southern California punishes teams by deducting points from their league standings when they accumulate fouls: 1 point for a yellow card (warning), 2 for a red card (expulsion); at 20 points a team loses 1 point in the standings, at 30 it loses 2 points, at 40 it is banned from the organization.

Leagues (or schools) can establish workshops to teach parents the rules of the game. This can help them understand the skills involved and the difficulty of the judgment calls officials have to make.

The Michigan High School Athletic Association has thought extensively about how to develop good sportsmanship among the high school athletic community: athletes, administrators, teachers, parents, the media. They give athletes a questionnaire about unsportsmanlike conduct and arrange a pregame meeting between opponents. The questionnaire is also given to athletes or coaches who are ejected from games and asks them to reflect upon their actions from several perspectives and to figure out how to change:

- Why do you think it is against the regulations of this school to behave as you did?
- Why is it important for high school student athletes and coaches to set good examples?
- What did you accomplish by your behavior, other than being ejected from the contest?
- Indicate a plan that will assist you in improving your behavior.

Earl Hartman, athletic director of Mount Pleasant–Sacred Heart High School, instituted pregame meetings between his team and their opponents. He suggests questions to ask the opposing players ("Do you want to play ball in college?" "What are your teachers and classes like?") and then lets the boys mingle. He describes the results:

Midway through the contest, an event occurred that made me declare this first experiment a success. I had witnessed several . . .

previous games in which . . . one of our talented players had pounded walls, shook his head, scowled or cursed over a missed shot or turnover. At one point, this player had taken a baseline jumper that was blocked out of bounds by the opposing center. As the player stepped back onto the court for the inbounds play, he patted the opposing center on the shoulder and nodded to say "Nice play." The opposition was no longer nameless and faceless, but rather a respected opponent who, at least in this one battle, had succeeded and was acknowledged and respected for it!

See www.mhsaa.com/services/kit.pdf for Michigan's full sportsmanship kit.

Cheating

Cheating would seem to be an issue with an obvious, black-and-white answer: Cheating is wrong. But in fact it's tricky, and the answer depends on a number of things. What exactly is cheating? Games are defined by rules; without rules, there is no game. But are the rules absolute? And how do we interpret those rules?

Deliberately lying — for example, about a line call during a tennis game without designated officials — is cheating. The same for tampering with equipment, such as smearing football jerseys with Vaseline so that the opposition players cannot hold their tackles. Both of these are acts of conscious, active commission transgressing explicit rules that depend for enforcement on a voluntary honor code. In other words, no official can be expected to notice or sanction such a transgression. So far, so good.

But is it cheating if the line official calls the ball the wrong way in your favor and your teammates closest to the line say nothing (an act of omission)? What about pushing in a basketball game: Is a little push okay? What about a hard push? What if a player pushes someone much larger than himself and can't materially affect the opponent's move? When does pushing become a foul? What if the refs are allowing some pushing, or at least allowing a forearm on the opponent's hip, even though neither is permitted by the rules? Who determines what's fair, what's too much, and what are the grounds for the decision? So the first issue is to decide what is cheating and what isn't. Unhappily, the answers aren't always clear.

Clear-cut cheating becomes a problem when winning becomes more important than anything else to some players — usually around age twelve. Before that, however, when the point is fun, team play, and learning new skills, these objectives converge more naturally with the idea of winning with honor, with pure sportsmanship.

Some parents encourage cheating, even when this entails a conscious decision to lie. They do this by explicitly counseling their children to cheat, or by not discouraging cheating and insisting that they win no matter what. They might do this because they believe their ticket to a college scholarship or big bucks from a pro tour are available only through their child's demonstrated prowess in sports. This is a bad decision. It helps to remember that in the long run, parents aren't doing the kid any favors by concentrating on winning today at the expense of long-term principles. The ultimate goal is to help the athlete become a happy, productive adult. Even parents who consider their circumstances desperate should assess the high toll cheating takes on their child's character, reputation, and prospective sports career.

Other parents encourage cheating because they believe that everyone does it and their child will be handicapped by the lack of an important life skill if she grows up not knowing how to "work the system." This kind of cheating is usually less clear-cut than conscious lying, falling more in the realm of "spin": trying to persuade the official that the opponent, not you, knocked the ball out of bounds, or that the opponents fouled you when they didn't. It is often argued that it's up to officials to do their job properly and players should get away with what they can — or at least they don't have to be so honorable as to sabotage their own chances of winning.

Players should be clear about what the rules are — what precisely is a foul or cheating, and what isn't. If they know the rules, sometimes they can use them to their own advantage without breaking them.

- The hidden ball trick: The first baseman "consults" with the pitcher and returns to first base with the ball. The pitcher walks back toward the pitching mound, the runner wanders off first base, and the first baseman tags him out. This is devious, completely legal, and works about once a season.
- In the old days of football, the offensive team would send fifteen players onto the field between downs. At the last allowable moment, four would run off. This strategy, which prevented the defense from anticipating and preparing for the play to be run, seemed so blatantly unfair that the NFL changed the rule to prevent "slow-motion substitution."
- A world-class rower observed that just before a particular starter would shout "Go," his Adam's apple bobbed up and down. This rower would start his oars with the Adam's apple and gain a valuable microsecond head start.

The bottom line on cheating: The question for parents and players shouldn't be "What can we get away with?" but "If someone did this to me or my team, would I be angry?" (Yes, it's hard to maintain this frame of mind, but try anyway.)

✳

Most of us do our best to train our children, through advice and example, to choose the path of long-term ethical behavior. We assume that those who choose sound moral principles over unearned victories and easy distortions of fact live happier, more fulfilling lives. But it's far from a sure thing that people whose primary values are acquisition, power, and winning, no matter what the cost, are troubled or unhappy in any way. So those of us who hope our children choose ethical behavior also hope that the children find internal satisfaction, because we recognize that the world often does not recognize or reward doing the right thing. In sum, we hope for the best.

I watched a soccer league championship game in which a player was red-carded (expelled) for excessive force, so that his team was to play a man down. The player sneaked back on the field, and when the opposing team finally got the attention of the ref, who began counting players, the red-carded player ran off the field, stripping off his jersey so that his number could not be recorded. Clearly this kind of cheating was habitual for the team, and when I asked around, I learned that the team (and its league) did in fact have a reputation for thuggishness.

Rectifying this type of situation requires more than one parent's complaint. Who is there to talk to? The coach is encouraging loutish behavior, and the league is doing nothing to rein the team in. Pull your kid off this kind of team. What will he learn from such people except that winning is more important than anything else and that cutting corners and getting away with whatever you can is the way to win? This kind of team doesn't believe in working to improve skills, or developing pride or satisfaction from doing one's best. It doesn't believe that fun is important.

Coming at cheating from a different direction, preparation or research into opponents is a good idea for teams and officials. If the ref or the opponents were familiar with the thugs' tactics beforehand, they would have noticed the illegal man on the field more quickly and could have gotten him off faster.

If Sports Are Good for Boys, They're Good for Girls, Too

In 1972, Congress enacted Title IX of the Education Amendments, which prohibits sex discrimination in any educational institution that receives federal funds. Most high schools, public and private, fall into this category.

Title IX revolutionized athletics. In 1997, twenty-five years after the law took effect, the American Association of University Women reported these results, not all positive:

Before Title IX
- Girls were 1 percent of all high school athletes. Fewer than 32,000 women competed in intercollegiate athletics.
- Athletic scholarships for women were virtually nonexistent.
- Athletic opportunities for female students frequently were limited to cheerleading.
- Female college athletes received only 2 percent of overall athletic budgets.

Progress to date
- Girls account for 40 percent of all high school athletes. Women are 37 percent of all college varsity athletes.
- Female athletes receive only 23 percent of athletic scholarship dollars, and 27 percent of athletic recruiting dollars.
- The number (percentage) of women coaches in college athletics has decreased, down to 48 percent from 90 percent in the 1970s.

Source: http://www.aauw.org/1000/title9bd.html

Few today argue that girls should not be allowed to participate in athletics if they want, but how does Title IX play out on the ground? The issue that is most prominent is the allocation of an institution's finite resources. Title IX requires males and females to receive the same benefits from participating in sports, and in high school, benefits include:

- Equipment and supplies
- Scheduling of games and practice times
- Travel arrangements
- Coaching
- Publicity and support services

Expenditures

Equitable benefits means that boys' teams can't get new uniforms every year while girls' teams use last year's, or that boys' teams consistently travel to games by air-conditioned coach while girls' teams consistently travel by yellow school bus. On the other hand, it does not mean that a school can't spend more money on boys' equipment. For example, the football team is larger than any other team and requires more equipment; boys' lacrosse (a contact sport) requires different and more equipment than girls' lacrosse (a noncontact sport). And if a girls' team is traveling five miles while the boys' team is going five hundred miles, then the difference in bus comfort might well be acceptable to the teams as well as to the Office for Civil Rights (OCR) of the U.S. Department of Education, which enforces Title IX. Still, the school can't spend money to launder the boys' uniforms but not the girls'. Similarly, a school can't spend significantly more time and money to recruit and hire a boys' coach than a girls' coach.

Scheduling

One very visible Title IX issue is scheduling. In many locales, boys' games are traditionally held on Friday night, so that girls' games are often played on a weekday night. Weekday nights mean that fewer parents and friends can attend (which is why Friday was chosen for boys' games in the first place). The OCR considers this a violation of Title IX. Convenient and popular times should be alternated between girls' and boys' teams. The same holds true for practice times. It is inequitable for boys' practices to be held right after school and girls' practices at 6 p.m., so that girls have to go home and return, or wait around for practice. And further, the boys can't always be given the big new gym to practice and play in while the girls consistently use the smaller, older gym.

Extras

Some issues are less evident. If a booster club or generous donor offers team jackets or new uniforms to a boys' team, the school must find a way to provide the same benefit to girls. Once the school accepts the funding, it belongs to the school and must be disbursed equitably. Furthermore, because more boys play school sports than girls do, allowing gifts to specific teams is likely to perpetuate historic inequities.

If cheerleaders or bands are provided for boys' events, they must also be provided for girls' events, because they are considered publicity services. (I personally don't understand this — isn't publicity meant to attract attention *before* an event, not during? Shouldn't cheerleaders and bands show up when attendance warrants? I don't see them at boys' golf or water polo events.)

Coed Teams

Girls must be allowed to try out for the boys' team if the school has no girls' team in that sport. They can be disqualified if they are too small or too weak to play (these reasons are considered non-gender-related) as long as the same standards apply to boys as well. On the other hand, boys are not allowed to try out for girls' teams if in aggregate, more boys play at the school than girls. These rules are based on the assumption of underrepresentation of girls in athletic activities. If that is not the case at a particular institution, however, my concern as a sports doctor is that boys will be allowed to play on girls' teams. In high school, this is a bad idea, because the difference in speed and muscular strength makes a boy's presence on the field dangerous for girls and will probably make a difference in the final outcome as well.

> ## Y'All Come Now
>
> At many schools, attendance at girls' games is sparse. One coach of a girls' softball team instituted Parents Day at the first home game. She sends home a note inviting all parents to come to the game and a postgame picnic, and reminds them to bring a camera. This event gets parents mingling right away, so they see that the games are fun and the sidelines are the place to be. She says that at her school, this strategy resulted in every player being represented by one or both parents at every game last year, a remarkable achievement.

Although data specifically on Title IX at high schools are not available, the Women's Sports Foundation estimates that currently 80 percent or more of all colleges and universities are not in compliance with Title IX. This is nearly thirty years after the legislation was enacted, and despite the fact that every school or district that accepts federal funds must appoint a Title IX compliance officer.

Today, all too often, when a coach or parent points out to the high school principal that the schedule or locker room assignments favor the boys over the girls, the principal will shake his head and cluck, "Come on, you're making a mountain out of a molehill." Administrators who react this way are not only violating Title IX, they are not considering what they would do if the shoe were on the other foot, a test that is the essence of fairness. The equitable distribution of resources is basic. It's one thing to be ignorant of the law, or Title IX, it's quite another to prevent compliance with the law. Everyone makes a mistake once in a while, but how people rectify their mistakes should be a significant measure of their success as a professional and as a human being.

If you feel your child's school is in violation of Title IX, you can first discuss it with the coach, athletic director, or principal, and if necessary, contact the school's Title IX compliance officer. Be sure to do your homework: Gather as much information as possible, and find out how many people agree with you and will stand up with you. It's always more effective to complain as a group than as an individual. You must also consider possible adverse consequences to your child. It may not be fair, but the children of parents who complain may be ostracized and bullied by their peers, and suffer retaliation from the athletic department or school. If you find the school's response unsatisfactory, you can also submit a complaint to the Office for Civil Rights, or you can file a lawsuit. While either of these actions may be the right thing to do, in either case you will almost certainly find yourself very unpopular in the school community, and your child may be the one to suffer the fallout. Consider whether the sacrifice is worth it, and how much support you have from the community.

Foul Ball: When Bad Things Happen to Good Sports

As many of us know too well, injuries are part of athletics. Serious injuries, ones that keep an athlete sidelined for a season or more, can be devastating to the player — and his family. Suddenly the focus of his life is gone. He feels a deep sense of loss: he misses the joy of playing and excelling, the camaraderie of his teammates, the recognition of his achievements from friends, peers, and interested adults. A high-level player may further lose his chance at a college athletic scholarship.

Many injured athletes suffer moodiness and depression, isolation, frustration, anger, bitterness. Short-term, goal-specific psychological counseling from someone trained to work with athletes is often a good idea, especially for kids whose identity is tied to being an athlete; parents should be alert and sympathetic to the child's need to talk to someone who can help them cope with the situation. Ask a sports medicine doctor for names if you should ever need a sports psychologist for your child or for yourself.

An athlete with a long-term or permanent injury needs to decide whether or not to stay involved in sports. He can coach, either at his own school or in an outside league. He can also volunteer to manage a team, or become the commentator at games or a sportswriter for the school newspaper. These activities are a productive way of staying involved and can be satisfying in their own right, or they might be a painful reminder of what the athlete is missing. It depends on the kid. (When injuries ended his career, Bill Walton became an excellent television sports commentator. But he was already a celebrity when this happened. Kids often become injured before being able to gain renown in their own community, and this is hard for them, because most everyone wants to earn respect by doing something well.)

Tutoring others can also be helpful. It's always good to feel useful, and seeing others in need helps one keep a sense of perspective.

In general, parents should always help their kids maintain a diversity of interests — church youth groups, art and music lessons, photography, journalism. Help your child stay curious about the world by listening to her questions and offering information or pointing her to resources about her interests. This is a good idea even if it is obvious to you and your friends that your child can pitch a 90 mph fastball and is destined to be a Division I All-American. At some point he will no longer be able to play, due to age, injury, or other circumstances. In any case, encourage your child to lead a full life even when playing sports full time.

Serious injury is extremely difficult for all concerned. There is no good or certain best way to handle it. Try to be patient and kind, and to bear in mind the final proportion of things.

Notes from a Mother

My daughter Alexandra has had two serious knee surgeries for soccer injuries. She tore her right anterior cruciate ligament (ACL) in the spring of her freshman year of high school, and her left ACL in the spring of her sophomore year. As Jordan Metzl told us after the first tear, "There are worse things that can happen to a kid, but basically, this sucks." (Dr. Metzl had his own ACL reconstructed while in medical school.) ACL tears are becoming all too common among athletes of all ages, and mostly among girls. To avoid feeling sorry for oneself, it sometimes helps to remember that even fifteen years ago, a torn ACL was career-ending. Now it's season-ending, which is bad, but the surgery is successful in 95 percent of cases; and the athlete returns to play.

For Alexandra, these injuries meant very painful surgery followed by four to six months of rehabilitation: physical therapy three times a week, three or more hours of home exercises every day, and, starting about a month after surgery, going to the weight room at school every day and working with a trainer on the weight machines or in the pool for underwater running. Twice. Two years in a row. It meant no summer camp, no summer community service, and, worst of all for a high school athlete, no playing soccer on her school team for two seasons, half her high school career.

This situation was particularly difficult for Alexandra during school. It was hard to leave her friends during free periods to go off to work with the trainer. It was harder to see her friends suiting up for games she couldn't play in. She missed having fun with the team, missed representing her school, missed the plaudits and attention that accrue to someone who does something very well.

She went to a few of her school soccer games and attended virtually all of her club team games, including overnight tournaments, even though she couldn't play. We all felt it was important for her to remain part of her club team. She had been a member since she was nine and was close to many of the girls. In her second injury season, her coach made her his assistant and had her speak to the girls in the halftime huddle of every game, thus giving her a genuine and useful role on the team. This was not simply a make-work position but a task to which she was well suited as a serious and analytical player with an understanding of tactics and field vision.

Her major soccer worry during rehab was that she would lose her skills. She didn't — but of course she didn't improve them either, since she lost two playing seasons. She did lose speed, however. As she said, "My feet don't work as fast." Watching others who had gone through the rehab process encouraged her to think that she would regain that speed, but it might take a year or more.

Alexandra also became a baseball fan while watching Yankees games with her father as she did her nightly exercises.

As a family, we tried not to spoil her too much, although I did notice that I bought her more clothes than I normally would, and we let her slack off on some of her chores because she would plead that she had no time due to her exercise schedule.

The summers were hard not only because her plans were disrupted (maintaining mountain trails in the Adirondacks and soccer camp), but also because most of her friends were out of town. Finding something useful to do helped a lot. The first summer, she was able to help with a medical research project and studied Chinese. The second summer, she tried to tutor younger kids but found this difficult to schedule between her physical therapy appointments and her home exercises. That second summer she also burrowed more into herself, just gritting her teeth to get through it a second time.

Friends came to visit after the surgery. They sent flowers, they brought us dinner. They made us go out to dinner when we sounded particularly frazzled. Her coach called and came to visit. We were so grateful to all of them.

The three of us spent a lot more time than usual just being together. We went to virtually every summer teen movie; we went shopping a lot; we went out to lunch occasionally; sometimes we cooked together. We also talked with each other much more than usual — about silly things, about weighty philosophical matters, such as how unfair it is that talent is distributed unevenly or how political bias impedes objective discussion, or about news items.

Best of all, her father and I read aloud to her for hours while she was doing her exercises. There's nothing like reading aloud and sharing the excitement, disasters, and triumphs of a great story. We read all of the Harry Potters (the first three twice), Philip Pullman's *Golden Compass* trilogy, Orson Scott Card's *Ender's Game,* Harper Lee's *To Kill a Mockingbird,* the James Herriot veterinarian books. We loved them.

Of course we fervently hope never to go through another such surgery and post-op period, and we cringe whenever we hear of another child (or adult) being seriously injured. But the lessons we came away with are that even a terrible period can produce happy, memorable moments to enjoy together with your child, and that what's really important in life is to spend time with family and friends.

Carol Shookhoff

Box Score

- Keep in mind the long-term development of your child.
- Help your child develop multiple interests.
- Learning to be fair and empathetic while being competitive is a particular benefit of sports.

Chapter 5

The Developing Athlete

ADOLESCENCE AND SPORTS

This chapter is about the many changes — physical, physiological, and psychological — in the developing teen's body, and how these changes affect sports performance.

The parents of thirteen-year-old Jeffrey brought him to my office because he had injured his hand during preseason football practice. Taking care of the injury was the easy part. After I diagnosed a fractured radius, the discussion turned to football. "I want him to quit playing football," said his mother. "Now that some of the boys have gotten big, they can really get hurt." "Mom, football is what guys do. Besides, you're not the boss of me," said Jeffrey. Rather than witness World War III erupt in my office, I used the opportunity to talk about the tremendous changes in the adolescent body that make this stage of development both unique and challenging.

Once parents survive the trials of raising infants and young children, families are essentially on autopilot until the teen years hit. As I explained to both Jeffrey and his parents that day, no life stage involves greater change than adolescence.

"Why do I have to come home at midnight?" "What do you mean I have to get off the phone?" "Why are you always criticizing me?" "You are so embarrassing. Why do you always say such stupid things?" These are only a few of the questions thrown at many a

Key Terms

Adolescent development. The overall process of changing from child to teenager — physically, emotionally, psychologically — which usually occurs between the ages of 9 and 16.

Female Athlete Triad. Three unhealthy conditions — anorexia (disordered eating), amenorrhea (absence of menstrual periods), and osteoporosis (low bone density) — that occur in some athletic females.

Growth plate. Found at the ends of most bones in a child and developing teen; made of cartilage, it is prone to injury because it is much softer than bone.

Physiologic development. Changes in the body's ability to tolerate longer and longer periods of exercise, measured by $VO_{2\,Max}$ (maximum oxygen extraction).

Psychological development. Changes in the psyche of the adolescent toward autonomy and independence that make a person unique and provide a sense of self.

Sexual development. The maturation of teens that prepares the body to reproduce, manifested in visible changes such as breast development in girls and facial hair and the deepening voice in boys; these visible changes are also called secondary sex characteristics.

Skeletal development. Changes in the growing skeleton, including muscles and bones, that parallel sexual development.

dumbfounded parent of a developing adolescent. No matter how often they are warned about the turbulence of the teen years, parents are always amazed when their children begin to question their rules, their behavior, their values, and the family balance of power.

From a sports medicine perspective, the challenges of adolescence are many. The preadolescent body is totally predictable. Children know how fast they can run, how far they can bend, how much power they can exert. They also develop a sense of their limits, usually determined by fatigue. The adolescent body changes very rapidly, and with these changes, a whole new set of issues comes up. As the body gets bigger, it also gets stronger and faster. The mind becomes more independent. This new creature seeks ways to express itself, to "try on" or rehearse being an adult in the big world, often to the consternation of her parents, all while trying to familiarize herself with a new body that she doesn't feel entirely in control of. For parents, understanding these points is essential to effectively parenting the teen athlete.

The Changes We See: Sexual Development

During puberty, the body changes very quickly. These changes, which include height, weight, and body contour, occur as the individual moves from being a child to an adult over a period of seven to eight years. These visible changes are also called sexual development and are largely the result of surging hormones — testosterone in boys, estrogen in girls. When these sex hormone levels rise, the body and the phone bill grow very quickly.

In general, puberty starts two years earlier in girls than in boys. Around age ten, a girl's brain begins to deliver a cascade of hormones: the hypothalamus, the "command central" part of the brain, begins secreting a hormone that causes the pituitary gland, also in the brain, to signal the ovaries to begin secreting estrogen, a powerful steroid hormone that causes the female body to increase its fat deposits as well as to begin other changes, such as breast development and hip widening. As the level of estrogen rises, girls' bodies change rapidly. In addition, girls also secrete small amounts of testosterone, the steroid hormone that causes muscle development. In boys, the same hormones from the hypothalamus and pituitary glands cause the testicles to begin secreting testosterone, a powerful steroid hormone that causes the male body to grow taller, stronger, and faster. In boys, testosterone levels rise dramatically during the beginning of puberty, and this makes the "growth spurt" very notice-able. Boys can shoot up six or seven inches in one year during times of peak growth. Not only do they get taller quickly, the testosterone effect makes muscles much stronger as well. For girls, this is why taking illegal anabolic steroids, which are similar to testosterone, can have dramatic effects. Even a little extra testosterone can make them stronger. The downside is that girls also develop facial hair, acne, and a deepening voice. When adolescent athletes start taking these substances to increase their growth, they can put themselves into "premature puberty," because the body reacts to the increased testosterone levels. Ironically, prepubertal male athletes who take anabolic steroids (an estimated 8 percent of high school athletes) will end up shorter and with smaller testicles than they would other-wise, because when puberty starts early, it ends early. (See Chapter 6 for more on steroids.)

The age of the onset of puberty is different for everyone and is largely determined by genetics. Boys generally start puberty around the same age as their fathers did, and girls around the same age as their mothers. While girls generally start two to three years before boys do, there is a large bell-shaped curve of distribution. Some girls start early (age nine) and some much later (age fourteen). Boys tend to start puberty around age twelve, but some can start as late as six-teen. Several studies have shown that girls who begin puberty early and boys who begin puberty late are at risk for persecution by other students in their class. Often these early and late bloomers feel they are at the center of unwanted attention, and some have difficulty recovering from this state.

Sex hormones go into action when a certain level of fat develops in the body. Thus, in the industrialized countries, with their better nutrition, the age of puberty has been dropping. Young athletes whose sports value low body-fat content, such as dancing and figure skating, generally experience the onset of puberty one to two years later than their peers do. At this time, we are not sure whether this delay has any harmful effects in the long term.

As these changes begin, a preadolescent who knew what his body could and could not do often finds himself having difficulty anticipating his body movements. A preadolescent soccer player, for example, having passed the ball hundreds of times before, knows exactly how much force is needed to make the ball travel at a usable speed to a teammate ten feet away. When his body contour changes, he will often lose this sense, and sometimes it can take several years to return, when he becomes more comfortable in his new body type. Parents need to anticipate these frustrations, and to point out that much of this teen awkwardness will diminish with age.

For parents, understanding the significant adolescent stages of growth, development, and change is important because size does not correspond with physical maturity. Skeletal maturity does not correlate with sexual maturity, so even if a kid is big, he might still have open growth plates. (I will discuss growth plates and their importance shortly, in the section on skeletal development.) The changes that we see, the changes of sexual development — based on secondary sex characteristics such as the appearance of pubic hair and breasts — are the easiest way to ascertain what stage of maturation a teenager is in.

The Changes We Don't See:
Physiologic, Skeletal, and Psychological

As the developing adolescent's body grows, the changes we see on the outside are paralleled by changes on the inside that greatly affect how far, how fast, and how long a young athlete can perform. Physiologic development is the changes happening inside the body that allow for longer periods of endurance exercise. Skeletal development is the changes that happen in the growing bones and muscles. Psychological development refers to the changes in the maturing mind.

Physiologic Development: The Growing Ability to Tolerate Exercise

Eleven-year-old Eliot loves basketball and plays all the time — on the playground and on the local organized team. He also knows when he has played long enough: when he's tired, it's easy to see that he needs to come out of the game. Sarah is a sixteen-year-old basketball player whom I've treated for a stress fracture. Unlike Eliot, who has fatigue as his end point, Sarah has far greater stamina. "It seems as if she never gets tired," her mother would say. "When she was younger, she wouldn't play nearly as much, but as she has gotten older, she keeps going and going, like the Energizer Bunny."

The differences between Eliot and Sarah are indicative of what happens when kids become teenagers. As they grow on the outside, their internal physiologic makeup changes significantly, greatly increasing the body's ability to tolerate endurance exercise.

What governs the athlete's endurance is oxygen. The more oxygen available, the more the body is able to generate energy, known as adenosine triphosphate (ATP), which means it can sustain exercise for longer periods of time. In sports medicine, the term $VO_{2\,Max}$ (maximum oxygen extraction) is the measure often used to gauge physiologic fitness, also known as physiologic potential. The $VO_{2\,Max}$ increases for each athlete as he goes through puberty because the heart, like all muscles, gets stronger as kids grow. As the heart muscle increases in strength, it pumps more blood, so that more oxygen is available (oxygen is carried in blood).

As kids become more physiologically fit, parents need to watch out that they aren't exercising too much, since they can run and play sports for longer periods of time. Adolescents like Sarah are much more likely to develop overuse injuries such as stress fractures as they go through puberty because body fatigue is a much less limiting factor. (See Chapter 8 for more on overuse injuries.)

Skeletal Development: The Growing Bones and Muscles

The changes to the developing skeleton (bones and muscle) are fascinating and occur rapidly over only a few years.

Susan, a twelve-year-old field hockey player, is going through adolescent development. As her body changes, she notices that she can run for longer periods of time without getting tired. When she stretches, however, she can no longer bend over and touch her toes, which she could easily do only a couple of years ago; now she has trouble reaching her shins. Yesterday at practice she rolled over on her ankle. She has come to my office because her pediatrician is worried that she has suffered a growth-plate fracture.

Susan exemplifies some of the common issues of the developing adolescent skeleton. Becoming stronger, taller, and faster makes her a better athlete, but also means her body is more prone to injury. Imagine a go-cart, which can go only 10 miles per hour, running into a wall. When it hits the wall, the damage to car, wall, and driver is minimal. Now change the go-cart to a Porsche, going over 60 miles per hour. When the Porsche hits the wall, or another car, the damage is much greater. When kids (go-carts) become teenagers (Porsches), the injury rate increases dramatically as the force and speed generated by stronger muscles come into play. Teenagers are at least ten times more likely to injure themselves during sports than children are.

The developing adolescent skeleton changes almost everything about how teens play sports. For example, Little League or peewee football leagues have very low rates of injury, but in junior high, the injury rate of football players and athletes in other sports climbs by 50 to 60 percent.

The Growth Plates

What makes the skeleton grow is *growth plates* (see Figure 1, page 112), plates of cartilage found at the ends of most bones in the body. In basic terms, the developing teen's bones grow longer during puberty, when the cartilage cells in the growth plates start reproducing very quickly. This occurrence is called the *growth spurt*, which usually lasts for two to three years. During this period of rapid growth, the growth plates are especially susceptible to injury. As we will discuss in Chapter 10, rolling over on the ankle is often a ligament injury in an adult, whose growth plates are closed, but is frequently a growth-plate fracture in a developing athlete. Growth-plate injuries are potentially very serious. If not recognized and treated properly, they can result in bones that stop growing. I have a patient whose anklebone stopped growing, with the result that one side of the ankle was longer than the other and the foot rolled inward. Her sports career was over, and she had to have surgery to correct the imbalance in length.

The growth spurt usually occurs around age ten in girls and age twelve in boys. When it begins is based on the stage of development a child is in. This means that two eleven-year-old girls can be in the same class, on the same team, but be at different stages of development, and hence different stages of skeletal growth.

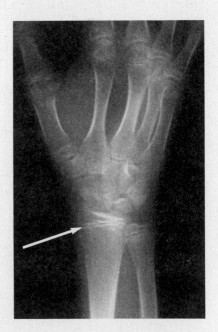

Figure 1.
X-ray showing a child's wrist with open growth plates. The arrow is pointing to one of the two main growth plates, which look clear in the X-ray because they are made of cartilage.

Flexibility

The reason the growth spurt affects sports performance so profoundly is that bones grow faster than muscles. Thus kids lose flexibility as they grow because the muscles are constantly trying to keep up with the growing bones. We have a saying in the office: "An adolescent can never stretch or study too much." This point is particularly relevant when kids go through their period of peak growth. If they skip the stretching, they continue to lose muscular flexibility and become much more prone to muscle tears (strains) as well as tendinitis (overuse injury of the muscle–tendon unit).

It is essential that adolescent athletes stretch their muscles at least three times a week to make up for this loss of flexibility that occurs as they grow. Teen athletes should stretch the major muscle groups — all of which are in the lower body: quads, hamstrings, calves — for twenty seconds without bouncing, just hold and a gentle stretch, with three repetitions of each group. Stretching is most effective when the muscles are a bit warm, say, ten minutes after a warm-up or a light jog. Coaches should build stretching into their practices.

Strength

The other element that changes significantly during skeletal growth is strength. Before puberty, girls and boys have relatively equal strength. As testosterone levels surge during adolescence, however, boys become much stronger than girls because testosterone, the male sex hormone, has a more significant effect on muscle development than estrogen, the female hormone, does.

This means coed contact sports such as soccer are safe before puberty, but around age twelve, the strength difference between boys and girls starts to become evident. When boys become stronger than girls, girls are at greater risk for injury when playing on the same team or same field because, in general, they aren't as strong.

The other important point about skeletal growth is the strength difference between kids at different stages of skeletal development.

Since strength increases as the skeleton matures, less-developed teens are more prone to injury than their teammates at a more advanced stage of development. For example, a junior varsity football team might be constituted of ninth graders, all thirteen or fourteen years old. Some of these young teens will be well into their growth spurt and will have muscles that are getting much stronger due to the effects of testosterone. Other teammates of the same age might be in the early stages of development and their muscles haven't yet become stronger.

Does this mean that all thirteen- or fourteen-year-old "late bloomers" should not play contact sports such as football? Of course not. Many parents have learned the following life lesson: If your teenager wants to do something, he will to do it whether you like it or not. Teens are remarkably industrious at figuring out ways to get around virtually every parental injunction. Rather than discourage your child from playing contact sports, emphasize the importance of preparing for the sports season. Lifting weights, even for kids as young as nine, can make a tremendous difference in how kids perform in sports and even in preventing injury. By lifting weights for six weeks before football season starts, an "underdeveloped," prepubertal thirteen-year-old can increase his baseline strength by 30 to 40 percent! We will discuss how to implement this type of program in Chapter 7. *Note:* Strength training, as its name implies, builds strength, not bulk.

Psychological Development: The Growing Self

Ashley, a nine-year-old ballerina, has seen me twice for tendinitis in her Achilles tendon. She loves to dance but also doesn't want to be injured, because then she can't participate in gym class and run around with her friends. Michael is a sixteen-year-old ballet dancer whom I have diagnosed with a stress fracture in his hip. Unlike Ashley, he wants to keep dancing at all costs, to be a professional dancer when he grows up. For Michael, injury is devastating, and he wants to focus all his energies on getting back to ballet class.

With Ashley and Michael, what's important to note is their respective stages of psychological development. Different people have different skill sets, and these interests and skill sets become evident during the teen years. Before puberty, the process of figuring out who you are and what you like to do isn't really apparent. Much like the developing physiology and skeleton, the growing psyche affects how kids see themselves and how far they are willing to push themselves. Ashley, for example, loves to dance but is also aware that a dance injury keeps her from her other activities. Michael, on the other hand, identifies himself as a dancer. He is undergoing the important stage of adolescence described by Erik Erikson as achieving *ego identity*. Essentially this means figuring out who you are and how you fit in to society, or balancing your own needs with those of others. (The task of finding where you belong in the larger world accounts for the overwhelming importance of the peer group in the lives of teenagers.) As kids grow, and as their bodies grow, so does their sense of identity, which means a sense that there is a dependable, ongoing core of values and abilities attached to an autonomous individual who is able to exert herself in the world in a meaningful way.

As teen athletes develop their own sense of who they are, they are much more likely to push themselves in sports to fulfill that identity. In my practice, I see many more overuse injuries, such as stress fractures, in adolescent athletes who are straining to reach the next level, to achieve the athletic identity they want for themselves, than in athletes who just play for fun. The more they strive, the more their bodies show signs of wear and tear.

For parents, the challenge, as always, is to be supportive and involved, but not controlling or pressuring. If a child is doing well in school and not getting injured in sports, it's probably fine to let him or her continue. But in cases such as Michael's, it's important not only to address the physical questions that arise, such as looking at bone density (stress fractures are often associated with lower bone density) and activity patterns (is the athlete doing too much exercise?), but also to consider the psychological questions as well. As they become teenagers and develop a sense of self, some kids form their primary identity around being an athlete. "I play soccer" is a very different statement than "I am a soccer player."

Sports Specialization in Growing Kids

Recently I gave a talk about kids and sports at a local school. One mother, in the second row, paid very close attention and took copious notes. During the Q&A, she asked, "My daughter Helen is eight years old and a competitive figure skater. Her coach doesn't want her to play basketball because she might be injured and playing will tire out the wrong muscles and impair her skating performance. What do you think?" This mother also wanted to know what sports her daughter could take up that would be safe and also improve her skating.

I told her I thought the coach was well intentioned but wrong. Young kids should not specialize in a single sport.

First of all, a child who plays only one sport does not develop physical responses to different physical situations; for example, doing nothing but skating limits the development of a variety of skill sets such as hand–eye coordination from hitting a baseball or shooting a basketball, or coiling, twisting movements from playing in the outfield. What kids gain from playing different sports is versatility and a rich movement vocabulary. Second, early specialization can lead to burnout and overuse injuries, especially when overzealous parents push kids to achieve. A young tennis player who wants to have fun can all too easily be transformed into a racquet-throwing brat who wants only to win. Third, a skater, whose sport revolves around solo performance and individual competition, will miss out on the invaluable experience of teamwork, group interaction, and social skills, important lessons to carry from the sports field to life. Finally, different body types are better suited to different sports. Someone who grows up to be short and lacking foot speed may not be a great basketball player but might do very well in ice hockey. But if he grows up playing only basketball, he may find the transition to another sport difficult because he doesn't have the moves.

It is true that specializing at a young age develops specific skills and muscles necessary to achieve at the top level. Most kids, however, just want to have fun and are not future Tiger Woodses. Moreover, the Woods family says that Tiger was the one who dedicated himself to golf; his parents did not push him. It's one thing if a child says "I want to be a great fencer and I will do whatever it takes to be great at fencing," and quite another if a child says "My coach says I should only skate and not play basketball."

For most kids, sports specialization should begin when they're teens, if at all. The American Academy of Pediatrics' policy statement on "Intensive Training and Sports Specialization in Young Athletes" (2000) says:

> Children involved in sports should be encouraged to participate in a variety of different activities and develop a wide range of skills. Young athletes who specialize in just one sport may be denied the benefits of varied activity while facing additional physical, physiologic, and psychologic demands from intense training and competition.

An unusually serious young child might want to focus on a particular sport (fencing, skating), but this is the exception, not the rule. The parent must pay very close attention to the child's reasons and behavior before deciding whether specialization is a good idea. Is the child unusually persistent when undertaking an interest? Does he characteristically fling himself into an activity with great enthusiasm and then tire of it a few months later? Why does he want to pursue this particular sport? Are his reasons sensible? Is he responding to the parent's pride in his achievements, hoping that specializing will bring him greater love and attention? And yes, even an eight-year-old should be able to give reasons for wanting to do something.

I told Helen's mother to let her play basketball.

Gender-Specific Developmental Concerns: Boys

Boys are active. They run, they jump, they're wild, and they can exhaust even the most energetic parent. With young boys, many parents think, "Just let me get them to the point where they're old enough to take care of themselves." For the most part, we turn out okay, though. One parent described the effort of trying to focus her adolescent son as like trying to harness Niagara Falls: If you can control the energy, you can light the entire city of Buffalo, but it takes time and effort. (My mom raised four sons, I'm not sure how she did it.)

When a sports experience is positive, the memories can last a lifetime; when the experience is difficult, it can last two lifetimes. It's much easier to be the parent of the quarterback or star soccer midfielder than of the benchwarmer. When failure occurs on the sports field, especially with boys, the parents, and more often the father, can sometimes feel personally responsible.

Effective parenting of the adolescent male depends on your ability to support your sons, regardless of athletic success. If you have a six- or seven-year-old hockey player at home, it's easy to emphasize the "just play for the fun of it" philosophy. When boys become teens, however, the emphasis invariably shifts toward winning. It's unrealistic to act like winning doesn't matter; it does matter, and you can lose credibility if you claim it doesn't. And winning becomes an issue during adolescence, because that's when kids begin to sort out their place in the world, comparing their own abilities to those of others. Winning versus losing is a handy measure.

As best you can, keep a sense of perspective. "Winning isn't everything, but it's sure easier than losing," and "You want to win with class and lose with class" are mottoes you can use when talking to a teenage son.

Boys' Specific Health Issues

After puberty starts, boys run faster, hit harder, and get hurt in sports about twice as often as girls do. Important health issues for the parents of adolescent boys include:

Protecting the Privates

In general, the high- and medium-contact sports require genital protection, and use should start around age ten. A good rule for parents is "As it gets bigger, it needs more protection." Some boys wear a jockstrap, an elastic-lined belt that holds the genitals in place during running. Boys playing sports such as football and soccer should try a *soft cup*, a protective device that offers more padding than hard protection and doesn't limit movement. In sports such as baseball, where contact injuries are more common, the traditional *hard cup* is a good idea. Some boys use a jockstrap to hold the protective cup in place, some just put the cup in their briefs and it stays put. What's important is that the protective cup is used and stays in place.

One fifteen-year-old in my practice was hit in the testicles trying to field a ground ball. He wasn't wearing a protective cup and suffered a ruptured testicle, which almost had to be removed. Teaching protective strategies before injuries happen is important; start discussing them with your son when he is nine or ten. (Also be sure to tell him that contrary to what he sees on television, he doesn't need to grab himself or spit to be a good baseball player.)

Protecting the Brain: Appropriate Headgear

Parents are more likely to think about helmets when they're required by a sport, and they're particularly aware of helmets in football. The football helmet needs to be snug, no more than one inch above the brow line, and the chinstrap should be snug. Make sure the football helmet is reevaluated each summer, before the season starts. Even at the ages of eight, nine, and ten, the head grows each year. Each football player needs a tight-fitting helmet to lessen the chance of head injury such as concussion. It's not okay to hand down the helmet from one brother to the next. To do your job as a parent, make sure it really fits.

Parents also need to focus on sports where helmets are optional but probably shouldn't be. Biking, rollerblading, skiing, and snowboarding are all sports that warrant mandatory helmet use. Each winter there are ten to fifteen deaths in the United States alone from skiing and snowboarding injuries to the brain. Helmet use would prevent many of these. It's important to make sure your kids are using helmets, even when others kids aren't. "It's not cool" is not an acceptable reason not to wear one. Have your kids use a helmet when they start these sports, and wearing one will become a habitual part of how they participate as they grow.

"Boy" Problems: Odors, Jock Itch, and Athlete's Foot

No discussion about the developing male is complete without mentioning the "boy" problems of body odor and skin infections such as jock itch. As the amount of testosterone increases, and as the secondary sexual characteristics such as underarm hair start developing, the odors emanating from males change distinctively. As boys get more hair, they also start to sweat more. An adorable athletic boy can quickly become a teenager whom parents might consider leaving on the porch for the night. Starting to use antiperspirants becomes important in the teen years (and hopefully beyond).

Tinea cruris (jock itch) and tinea pedis (athlete's foot) are two common fungal infections that become yet more common as boys become sweaty teens. Athletic attire such as running shorts and hockey gear are perfect habitats for fungi that thrive in a warm, damp environment. As boys become teens, they often need to change their hygiene habits. This includes making sure that athletic clothes dry out between uses, and that they are washed with greater frequency. If boys start getting itchy areas in the feet or groin, they need to try to keep the area dry; frequent use of a drying agent such as baby powder or one of the antifungal sprays available in drugstores is helpful.

Gender-Specific Developmental Concerns: Girls

The benefits of sports for girls extend off the field and have done much to change the way girls socialize. It used to be that only boys were given the chance to develop team-building and leadership skills, which often carried over into the classroom and the work environment. Boys thus tended to dominate the classroom discussion and took all the high-power jobs after college. Today, girls, playing in an equal-access world of sports, are learning about group dynamics and leadership in the ways boys always have. This has been terrific for them, and will change the way the girls of today interact with their daughters in the future.

In their parents' generation, most "serious" athletes were males, so that today the family's athletic tone for girls is often still set by fathers. But the idea of girls in sports is in many ways still new; there's a steep learning curve for dads as well as their daughters. "Every time I watch her play basketball, I'm so nervous I feel like my heart is going to jump out of my chest," one father told me. "I just want her to do well so she feels good about - herself. And she's only on the fourth-grade basketball team." When fathers learn that female athletics is every bit as competitive as the male version, they often get very involved in their daughters' sports careers. Mothers, whatever their own athletic history, are certainly getting into the act as well and can play an important role in the athletic lives of their daughters. The ideal situation for girls is one where both parents are involved, watching games and learning about the sport(s) their daughters participate in.

Girls' Specific Health Issues

"Female Athlete Triad"

Jenna, a sixteen-year-old cross-country runner who is nationally ranked and is also a great student, came to see me because of a stress fracture, which occurs when too much stress is placed on bone (sometimes from too much activity), and sometimes because the bone density is low (thinner bones tend to break easier). After diagnosing the fracture, I began to ask Jenna questions about her caloric intake and menstrual cycle. She told me that she has always been a picky eater, hates milk, and had not yet begun to menstruate. Taking care of Jenna involves not only treating her stress fracture, but also talking to her and her parents about the female athlete triad.

The female athlete triad is a serious health problem that we are seeing with increasing frequency. Its three components are anorexia (insufficient caloric intake), amenorrhea (absence of menstrual periods), and osteoporosis (decreased bone density).

Girls who are serious athletes need calories. Without enough food intake, they begin to develop a nutritional deficiency and begin to lose body fat. When body fat drops below 16 or 17 percent, girls can start to develop amenorrhea, which comes in two types: primary, meaning they don't get their period by age sixteen, or secondary, meaning their period stops for more than six months after they have started menstruating. When girls are amenorrheic, their ovaries don't make an egg and their estrogen level begins to drop, since egg production stimulates estrogen production. The last of the triad, osteoporosis, means weakening of the bones. There are two types of bone cells: osteoblasts, which are responsible for making bone, and osteoclasts, which break bone down. Normally they function in balance, allowing bodies to constantly upgrade or strengthen the bones. In girls with low estrogen, however, the two types of bone cells fall out of balance and the bones start to break down. (Osteoclast activity is restricted by estrogen, so when estrogen levels are low, the osteoclasts run wild; this is also why postmenopausal women take estrogen replacement to prevent osteoporosis.)

Parents need to be aware of this scenario, particularly with girls involved in sports such as running, dancing, and figure skating, where being thin is mandatory for success. Important questions to keep track of include:

- Has my daughter started her period by age fifteen?
- Has my daughter had a stress fracture?
- Is my daughter taking in enough calcium (she needs about 1500mg a day, about three eight-ounce glasses of milk)?
- Does my daughter look too thin?

If your daughter has not menstruated by age fifteen, or has had a stress fracture, or is not taking in enough food or calcium, please discuss this with her physician, either a pediatrician or an adolescent medicine specialist. Increasingly, we are using a test called a DEXA (dual energy X-ray absorptiometry) to screen for osteoporosis; it is painless and uses very low doses of X-ray to evaluate bone density. Since bone density peaks around age thirty-one, the bone your daughter is making as a teenager is very important in determining her eventual bone density in middle and old age. Several studies have shown that former ballet dancers who manifested the female athlete triad as adolescents have lower bone density as adults. When they are sixty and seventy, they will be at higher risk of suffering fractures of the hip and spine. So prevention is key. Talking about this with your teenager is important and can help make her aware of the consequences of eating properly, both now and in her future.

Proper Support: Sports Bras

A very helpful invention of the past ten years is the sports bra, which supports the ligaments at the top of the breasts (Cooper's ligaments) and thus prevents the breasts from sagging later in life. They should be worn during exercise once breasts start to develop. Sports bras should fit tightly but not restrict motion. Girls with large breasts who want more support can use two bras, one on top of the other.

ACL Injuries

As described earlier, Alex is a sixteen-year-old soccer player who has had two reconstructions of her anterior cruciate ligament (ACL), one on each knee. Both times, while taking the ball up the sideline for her club team, she cut to elude a defender and heard a *pop* in her knee. She fell over, with no contact from her opponent, and her knee began to swell immediately so that she couldn't put weight on it. Before she could have surgery, she had to rehab her knee for about a month to regain full mobility. After surgery, she spent three to five hours a day for four months rebuilding her leg muscles.

An ACL tear is a big-deal injury. ACL injuries in women are currently being studied around the world. Boys tear their ACLs as well, but at this point, we know that female athletes, especially those involved in sports that involve twisting or cutting movements such as soccer or basketball, are at least three to four times more likely to tear their ACL than boys are. Chapter 10 covers the theories explaining this disparity, but the real answer is that we still aren't sure why.

What's important here is prevention. If you have a daughter who plays basketball, soccer, or field hockey, have her work on strengthening her hamstring muscles. Girls' hamstring muscles are usually much weaker than their quadricep muscles; boys' quadricep and hamstring strength is more balanced. Again, we don't know why this is. The end result, however, is that when a girl stops or starts quickly, the femur (thighbone) is pulled forward by the quadricep and the hamstring is less able to resist this force. The ACL sits between the femur and the tibia (shinbone), and when these bones are forcefully pulled apart, the ligament is torn.

Parents, coaches, and doctors are all concerned with preventing ACL injuries. Thus far, the only prevention programs that seem at all promising are those that include isolated hamstring strengthening. So, encourage your daughter to start on such a program; at the very least, as my grandmother used to say, "It can't hurt."

Hamstring Strengthening

Have your daughter lie on her stomach with her legs out straight. A helper then places a towel over one heel and grasps both ends. Have her bend her leg, against resistance, pulling her heel toward her buttocks. Do three sets of 15 repetitions on each side. Do this simple exercise a minimum of four times a week for six weeks. It can make the hamstrings stronger and reduce the risk of ACL injury.

Your child can also do this exercise by herself with a 10- or 15-pound ankle weight. While lying on knees and elbows, with one leg extended, she should slowly do three sets of 15 repetitions on each side.

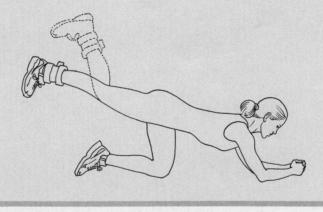

Adolescence seems to happen almost overnight. The changes it entails dramatically affect how kids exercise, what they are able to do, and how long they are able to do it. By understanding the major points of adolescent development, parents can anticipate some of the issues that become important as kids grow. Parents need to be aware of certain gender-specific issues for their sons and daughters.

Box Score

- Understand the changes your growing teens are experiencing.
- During your children's adolescence, your must be more alert to the increased risk of sports injuries and know how to prevent them.
- Make sure boys are outfitted with the proper equipment.
- Make sure girls are eating properly, especially if they are in sports that require them to be thin.
- Make sure girls strengthen their hamstrings if they play twisting or cutting sports.

Chapter 6

Nutrition and Nutritional Supplements

THE GOOD, THE BAD, AND THE UGLY

This chapter covers what to eat to promote growth and performance,
and what to avoid to prevent health risks.

Why do we eat? Because we're hungry, food tastes good and makes us feel better, and meals can be pleasurable social occasions. Why do we need food? This question is the basis of the field of nutrition. We need food to grow properly and have enough energy to do what we want. Nutrition can be divided into four basic areas: healthy physical growth, performance enhancement, weight control, and preventive eating (eating to avoid future diseases).

Now, when your children are growing, is the time to establish proper eating habits for long-term good health.

Nutrition for Growth and Energy

A balanced diet — that is, a diet based on variety and whole-someness — is essential to healthy physical growth and energy on demand. This means eating primarily complex, or starchy,

Key Terms

Carbohydrate. One of the three energy-producing nutrients (along with protein and fat). Carbohydrates are either complex or simple.

Complex carbohydrate. Starchy carbohydrate found primarily in plants and consumed as cereals, breads, other whole grains, and potatoes.

Simple carbohydrate. Sugars, such as candy, sugared cereal, and just plain sugar.

Fat. One of the three energy-producing nutrients; the body needs very little fat as a nutrient and stores it for long-term energy.

Glucose. The sugar that carbohydrates break down into. It is readily absorbed into the bloodstream.

Glycogen. The stored form of glucose, found mostly in the liver but also in muscle. Glycogen is broken down into glucose for use during exercise.

Protein. One of the three energy-producing nutrients, available from plants as well as animals. The body uses protein to build and repair muscle. Most adolescents don't get enough protein in their diet.

Vitamins and minerals. Nutrients that provide no energy but that are essential in helping energy-producing nutrients function properly in the body. The body cannot produce certain vitamins and minerals on its own and needs to ingest them from food sources.

carbohydrates such as cereals, breads, and other whole grains, as well as fruits and vegetables (as distinct from eating simple, sugary carbohydrates), accompanied by a small portion of meat or fish. That's right, a healthy meal dominated by complex carbohydrates is the opposite of what most of us picture when we think of dinner. Protein, along with essential vitamins and minerals present in dairy foods, fruits, and vegetables, is also necessary for proper growth. (Essential vitamins and minerals are nutrients your body cannot produce on its own; you need to get them from food.)

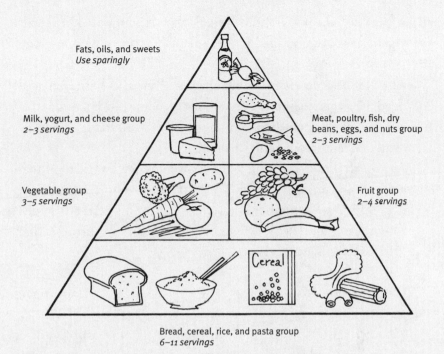

Figure 2.

The Food Guide Pyramid. *Source:* U.S. Department of Agriculture

Plan your family's meals by consulting the U.S. Department of Agriculture Food Guide Pyramid, which illustrates how much of each food group to eat every day, but bear in mind several important points.

• The USDA serving sizes are very small. If you give up on the RDAs (recommended daily allowances) because six to eleven servings of the carbohydrate group seem impossible to attain, remember that the USDA considers one slice of bread one serving; so is ½ cup of cold cereal (the size of half a tennis ball). For the dairy and protein categories, one serving of cheese is the size of four dice (yes, dice, as in board games), and one serving of meat means a portion the size of a deck of cards. (The nutritionists' size equivalents are very courageous: carnivores fall into a faint just thinking about a steak as small as a deck of cards; vegetarians are outraged by the idea of cutting a cow into tiny pieces.)

• The USDA-recommended number of servings is based on adult needs. It is also based on very broad generalizations. Individual needs range widely from child to child, adolescent to adolescent, and even from adult to adult.

• As a general rule, growing teenage athletes need more food than adults do — anywhere from 1,500 to 3,000 more calories a day, depending on a number of factors, including gender, height, weight, and activity level. They also need more protein than their couch potato peers do.

Everything we do — from reading this page, to turning over in our sleep, to swinging a baseball bat — requires energy. Energy is supplied by the calories from food, mostly from carbohydrates (which are digested into glucose) and a little from fat. Extra carbohydrates, whether eaten as sugar (fruit juices, honey, candy) or starch (grains, cereals, potatoes), are stored in the muscles and liver in the form of glycogen. Depending on the type of activity involved, the body will use different energy stores. When engaging in high-intensity exercise requiring short bursts of energy — such as weight lifting, sprinting, racing, soccer, football, basketball — the body will rely primarily on glycogen (the stored form of glucose) for energy. During low-intensity exercise such as walking, the muscles burn mostly fat for energy. Furthermore, during endurance activities such as cycling and marathon running, which require a constant supply of energy over a long period of time, the body will start out burning carbohydrates and end up dipping into fat stores when muscle glycogen is depleted.

An athlete's energy (calorie) needs are determined by his individual goals. A defensive football player may want to bulk up so he can hit harder, while a wrestler may want to lose a few pounds to make a lower weight class.

Calories

A calorie is the unit of energy needed to raise the temperature of 1 gram of water 1 degree Centigrade. When we refer to calories in food, we are talking about the amount of heat needed to break down or metabolize the food. Calories can also refer to the amount of energy the body uses (as in a person's "daily caloric needs"). All foods have a caloric value, determined by the amount of protein, carbohydrate, and/or fat they contain. Different nutrients have different caloric densities. Carbohydrates and protein, for example, each supply 4 calories per gram, while fat supplies 9 calories per gram, more than double the calories in 1 gram of carbohydrate or protein. No wonder fatty foods are so fattening!

To complicate matters further, foods that seem similar in type and caloric value may offer very different nutritional value. Take fruits, for instance, which are all high in energy-packed carbohydrates. One cup of cubed cantaloupe provides about 60 calories and is an excellent source of vitamin A and potassium. A 60-calorie cup of honeydew melon, however, supplies little to none of a child's recommended daily allowance of the free radical–fighting antioxidant vitamin A. So you might say that for the same 60 calories, cantaloupe has more bang for the buck than honeydew, nutritionally speaking.

Some Foods High in Complex Carbohydrate

Bananas, bagels, fruit, rice, raisins, dried apricots, pasta, baked potato, fruit yogurt, dried beans, English muffins

What to Push with Your Kids

The body also needs fiber as an integral element of a healthy, energy-sustaining diet. Fiber serves many important functions in the body, and a diet high in fiber can help maintain regular bowel movements (preventing constipation), reduce cholesterol, and regulate blood sugar levels. Furthermore, a wealth of scientific research over the years strongly indicates that a high-fiber, low-fat diet is effective in fighting cancer and heart disease.

Different grains (breads, cereals, pastas) have different amounts of fiber. To illustrate the variable nutritional value of different grains, let's look at that ever-popular snack, peanut butter and jelly. A peanut butter and jelly sandwich on two slices of white bread provides little to no fiber, while the same sandwich on 100 percent whole-wheat bread may supply anywhere from 4 to 6 grams of dietary fiber, almost 25 percent of a person's minimum daily goal (25 to 35 grams of fiber a day). That is not to mention the abundance of B-complex vitamins and disease-fighting phytonutrients also present in whole-wheat bread.

There's no way to tell about fiber without reading the label. Don't worry too much about soluble versus nonsoluble fiber; the important thing is to get some fiber into the system. Choose cereals with 5 or more grams of fiber per serving and breads with at least 2 grams of fiber per slice. Experiment with different breads, such as seven-grain, oatmeal, branola. Try whole-wheat pasta instead of regular. Whole-grain breads and cereals often have a sweet, nutty flavor some kids like. Pretzels even come in a honey whole-wheat variety, and they are excellent.

No matter how much you know about nutrition, however, the fact is that some kids will eat anything you put in front of them, while others are picky, and what they are willing to eat depends on what day of the week it is. In general, to ensure that your child is getting all his essential nutrients, work on achieving:

- **Balance** between different types of foods
- **Moderation** in high-sugar and high-fat foods (fast food, fried foods, cakes, cookies, candy, soda)
- **Variety** among fruits and vegetables. Keep in mind that carbohydrates such as those found in whole grains, fruits, vegetables, and low-fat dairy products are the body's preferred fuel source.

Note that foods need not always be fresh. Canned fish (tuna, salmon, sardines) offers as many nutrients as fresh-caught fish; frozen vegetables have as many nutrients as fresh, and possibly more when vegetables are out of season.

Here's what to try to get your kids to eat:

- Starchy carbohydrates, especially whole-grain breads and cereals, brown and wild rice, whole-wheat pasta (for fiber)
- Dark-colored vegetables, especially leafy green, dark green, and orange vegetables such as spinach, broccoli, kale, collards, zucchini, carrots, sweet potatoes
- Citrus fruit or other food high in vitamin C (oranges, grapefruit, strawberries, broccoli, potatoes, green and red bell peppers, kiwi)
- Two cups of low-fat or skim milk, fortified soy milk, or two servings of low-fat yogurt or cottage cheese daily (for calcium)
- Grilled, baked, steamed foods instead of fried
- Protein sources low in saturated (bad) fats, such as chicken and turkey without the skin; fish; beans; tenderloin of pork; veal; low-fat or nonfat yogurt, cottage cheese, and milk; nuts; tofu and other soy-based products.

Your success in meeting these nutritional goals may depend on the age and preferences of the individual child. When children are small, parents have much more control over what they eat because kids eat most of their meals at home. When they're teens, however, they're gone all the time and seem to subsist on junk food — even athletes, who ought to know better.

Here are a few suggestions:

- *The family dinner.* The family dinner is an endangered species in the era of the two-earner family with an athlete going to practice every day. But try to have at least three or four a week. The family dinner is an important time for parents and kids to be together and talk. It's also a meal when parents can make sure a variety of nutritious foods is available to their child, and they can hope he remembers the example and chooses to eat a green vegetable once in a while when he's out with his friends or off at college.

- *The twenty-four-hour food diary.* Ask your child to write down everything she eats for twenty-four hours as an experiment. She might find the percentage of good food versus junk food eye-opening, and seeing the list in black and white is often a concrete visual stimulus to eat properly, or at least *more* properly. Many student athletes avoid abusing controlled substances because they understand that bad chemicals will impair their performance; the same rationale might induce them to eat a healthier diet than they would ordinarily choose for themselves.

- *Make healthy food convenient.* Cut up snacks (fruit, carrot and celery sticks, cheese) and peel them if necessary before the kids get home so good food is easy to eat and available the minute they want it. This is especially helpful for teens, who live in the moment. When they're hungry, they don't want to wait, they don't want to work, they just want to eat. Also make healthy snacks transportable (bagel with cream cheese, PB&J sandwiches cut into quarters, a slice of quiche, raisins, dried apricots) so kids can take them with them and not rely on the ubiquitous snack trucks.

- *Build on what your child likes.* Experiment with dishes you know she likes to see what you can add. Try sneaking tofu or grated carrots into spaghetti sauce or the tuna salad you mix for sandwiches. If she likes sausage, try turkey sausage. Instead of chocolate cake, see if she'll eat carrot cake or banana bread. If she devours chips, see if she'll switch to pretzels. If she eats pita bread, try whole-wheat pita. Don't, of course, force your kid to eat something she dislikes. If these experiments fail, so be it. You've done your best.

- *Keep offering vegetables.* If you can make eating vegetables a habit with your children, you will have done one of the best things possible for their long-term health. Try different vegetables in different forms: For example, spinach can be eaten raw in salads or cooked and pureed in soups and dips. Roasting vegetables brings out their sweetness (beets and cauliflower are delicious roasted). Try adding raisins to greens or orange juice to broccoli. Try different salad dressings, different gazpacho recipes. Put out colorful baby carrots, cherry tomatoes, and crisp string beans and bell pepper strips with a low-fat-yogurt–based dipping sauce while the kids are doing homework. Experiment with tabbouleh (aka parsley salad) until you find a version your child will eat.

- *Try different low-fat, low-salt, low-sugar foods and snacks.* This is a tough battle to win with teens because most of these foods just don't taste good. Try potato chips and tortilla chips that are baked instead of fried. You can cut whole-wheat pita bread into triangles, brush them with a little olive oil, garlic powder, and dried oregano, then bake them in the oven until crisp; they make a delicious snack. So do dried fruit and cereal or home-made low-fat granola.

If all else fails, consider consulting a nutritionist (or registered dietitian) who has worked with young athletes. Ask your pediatrician or other parents who have seen nutritionists for recommendations. I also recommend this for kids who want to achieve optimal nutrition, and for kids who are restricting calories to improve sports performance, usually runners, dancers, and gymnasts. Nutritionists can help devise healthy strategies for kids and give good guidelines for parents.

Remember the Basics

Your child needs breakfast. All the body's energy stores are depleted by morning and need replenishment. Without breakfast, she's more likely to faint, have headaches, or be lethargic and unable to concentrate. Try to include a little protein with breakfast such as low-fat milk, yogurt, or cottage cheese, egg, or peanut butter.

Your child also needs sleep, more than eight hours a night. Maybe he needs to cut out television altogether, or to "power nap" in spare moments (preferably not in class).

One Recipe: Banana Smoothie

I'm including this because so many kids like it, and it's fast, easy, and good for them.

> 1 carton yogurt (plain, with fruit, 8-ounce size or smaller —
>   it doesn't matter)
> ½ the yogurt carton of milk (whole, low-fat, etc.)
> 1 banana
> 1 heaping tsp. strawberry jam

Throw into the blender and whir.

My athlete has become a vegetarian — is this safe?

Carefully planned vegetarian intake can provide adequate amounts of the protein, carbohydrates, minerals, and vitamins that a young athlete needs to grow properly and perform well. Teenagers, however, tend to be creatures of impulse and avoid planning or sticking to a plan. In addition, teen athletes often have full schedules and are likely to end up eating snacks or fast food on the run. I advise parents and vegetarian athletes to consult a registered dietitian to be sure nutrition doesn't become a problem.

Should my child take vitamins?

If your child is eating a good, balanced diet, he won't need pills. On the other hand, a daily multivitamin benefits most people, isn't harmful, and may be reassuring to both you and your child. NOTE: Massive doses of single vitamins, however, can be harmful.

If your child is a vegetarian (no animal products except eggs and dairy) or vegan (no animal or dairy products at all), she may not be getting enough B12, iron, or zinc. In this case, a multivitamin and perhaps a B-complex supplement may be recommended. Consult your child's doctor.

Does my daughter need extra iron?

Iron is an essential nutrient for everyone, but once girls begin to menstruate, they need more iron than their male peers do to compensate for menstrual losses. Iron deficiency (insufficient iron stores in the blood) impairs athletic performance and is usually caused by a poor diet. It is more prevalent in females than males and is notable among cross-country runners. In addition, female athletes who are vegetarians are at greater risk for anemia, which is more serious than iron deficiency.

Anemia, a low red-blood-cell count, occurs when the body is unable to make red blood cells because it lacks iron. Red blood cells carry oxygen. With fewer red blood cells, anemic athletes get tired easily. If you have a female athlete who seems to tire easily and isn't getting a lot of iron in her diet, be sure to have her discuss this situation with her doctor. (Adolescent-medicine physicians specialize in teens and provide an environment where these concerns can be raised comfortably.)

Female athletes should generally have a blood test about once a year, but each individual should discuss the frequency with her doctor. If their iron levels are low, they should eat iron-rich foods — red meat, liver, poultry, fish, oysters, clams, beans, spinach, tofu, iron-fortified cereals, prune juice, enriched pasta, molasses, brewer's yeast, wheat germ — or take an iron supplement under the supervision of their doctor. This will remedy the immediate condition, but the doctor will often look into the underlying cause to be sure that low iron levels are not related to more serious health issues.

Nutrition to Enhance Performance

The Pre-Game Meal

Pre-event meals are intended to stave off hunger, which impairs focus, and to store enough energy to keep the athlete going. Carbohydrates are the basis for energy in endurance sports as well as power sports. The body takes twenty-four to forty-eight hours to restore the muscle fuel (glycogen) supplied by carbs, so one or two days before the event, the athlete should begin to get about 65 to 70 percent of calories from carbohydrates at each meal.

Shortly before the game, a light meal should be eaten to prevent hunger. These foods should be easy to digest. That means low-fat, low-fiber food that the athlete knows his system can tolerate. The day of an event is not the time to try a new food.

The timing of meals and snacks will depend on the individual; athletes should keep track of what and when they prefer to eat before an event. Portions should get smaller, however, as game time approaches. If he likes, the athlete can consume a small quantity of carbohydrate just before competing — a banana, a few crackers, a cup of sports drink.

If your child prefers to skip breakfast when she has an early-morning game or competition, a high-carbohydrate snack at bedtime the night before (such as a bowl of cereal and milk or a couple of pieces of toast with peanut butter) can help ensure that an athlete is not energy-depleted the morning of the event.

Food during the Event

A small amount of carbohydrates during an endurance event lasting more than sixty to ninety minutes can delay fatigue. Eating 40 to 60 grams of carbohydrate (about 100 to 300 calories) per hour of exercise can help maintain blood sugar levels. To give you an idea, 150 calories of carbohydrate is equivalent to a large banana, two 12-ounce bottles of a sports drink (at 50 calories per 8 ounces), half a bagel, some sports bars, or a homemade sports cocktail of 8 ounces orange juice mixed with 8 ounces water.

Food after the Event

Muscle glycogen (energy) is most effectively restored by consuming carbohydrates within thirty minutes after vigorous exercise, fol-

Pre-Exercise Meal Guidelines		
3 or more hours before	**2–3 hours before**	**1–2 hours before**
Fruit or vegetable juice, sports drink	Fruit or vegetable juice, sports drink	Fruit or vegetable juice, sports drink
Fresh fruit	Fresh fruit	Fresh fruit (low-fiber, such as honeydew, watermelon)
Breads, bagels, crackers, English muffins	Breads, bagels, crackers, English muffins	
Peanut butter, lean meat, low-fat cheese		
Low-fat yogurt (regular or frozen)		
Pasta with tomato sauce		
Cereal with low-fat milk		

Source: Suzanne Nelson Steen, D.Sc., R.D., and David T. Bernhardt, M.D., "Nutrition and Weight Control," in J. Andy Sullivan, M.D., and Steven J. Anderson, M.D., eds., *Care of the Young Athlete* (American Academy of Orthopaedic Surgeons and American Academy of Pediatrics, 1998).

lowed by yet more carbs two hours later. You build up more glycogen by eating sooner than you get by eating the same amount later in the day.

Fluids (Hydration)

The human body is approximately 60 percent water. Body water transports oxygen and nutrients to the muscles and carries away lactic acid that builds up in the muscles during activity, often inhibiting performance. It also transports the heat generated by exercising muscles to the skin surface, where it is dissipated through sweat. The sweat then evaporates and cools the body to stabilize core temperature. Sufficient water in the body is thus essential to optimal performance, as well as good health. Even slight dehydration can impair athletic performance, and as little as 5 percent dehydration can cause cramping, chills, and nausea. More acute dehydration can result in dizziness and fatigue. And an athlete doesn't need to feel thirsty to be dehydrated.

Did you know that one of the most common causes of gastrointestinal complaints in runners is dehydration? As a runner, when I'm dehydrated I feel sluggish and slow, but just a few glasses of water can improve my time. Recent research suggests that Americans are chronically dehydrated. This is just another reminder that we should all drink more water every day.

When someone becomes extremely dehydrated, he risks severe medical complications. Several studies have shown that muscle strains are more likely to develop with dehydration. So proper hydration is also important for injury prevention.

Young athletes should drink plenty of fluids to compensate for their fluid losses, even if they aren't thirsty. This is especially true for prepubescent children who don't yet sweat much and do not tolerate temperature extremes as well as adults can. Starting children with effective hydration techniques when they are young encourages effective hydration behavior throughout their sports career.

Fluid Intake Guidelines

12–24 hours before event	During event	8 hours after event
Drink enough so that the urine is almost colorless.	Drink ½ cup to 1 cup (4 to 8 ounces) of water or sports drink every 15 to 20 minutes depending on tolerance (not juice or carbonated soda — they have too much carbohydrate for easy absorption).	Drink 2 to 4 cups (16 to 24 ounces) for each pound of weight lost during exercise.

Be aware of the early signs of dehydration, which include tiring easily, irritability, and a sudden decline in performance. Kids can become dehydrated before they feel thirsty, so it's important that they have regular drink breaks.

A coach should always allow a break when an athlete says she's thirsty and never withhold water privileges as a punishment for infractions or lack of effort.

Fluids at Extreme Temperatures

Temperature alone is not a reliable guide to the amount of fluid an athlete needs. Most parents recognize the risk of dehydration when the weather is hot and humid, but dehydration can also occur in cool or cold weather. Furthermore, wind and humidity need to be considered in conjunction with temperature when assessing the environmental threat to maintaining the athlete's core body temperature.

The 80/80 Rule: If the temperature is higher than 80 degrees and the humidity is higher than 80 percent, it is very difficult to dissipate sweat, increasing the risk of dehydration and heat illness. When both heat and humidity are high, check with the athletic trainer or coach and mention the risk of dehydration. Coaches should be aware of the signs of heat illness — cramping and headaches — especially with athletes who have had heat exhaustion before, because they are more likely to develop it again. In extreme conditions, players should drink a cup of water every twenty minutes and be given timeouts to rest in the shade. At very high levels of play, monitoring daily weight loss is a good idea.

An elevated core body temperature is a medical emergency. Warning signs include headache; fatigue; chills; tingling in the arms and back; cool, moist skin; weak, rapid pulse; dizziness. Any athlete exhibiting these symptoms should leave the field, sit in the shade, sip cool fluids, and call for medical assistance.

Commercial Products

Should My Child Drink Water or a Sports Drink?

Water is an inexpensive, excellent fluid to hydrate the body, but if young athletes are more willing to drink a sports drink because of the flavor, let them. After an hour of activity, sports drinks are recommended because they replace salts as well as carbohydrates and can prevent hyponatremia (low blood sodium).

What about sports bars?

To most people, "energy" means more power, the ability to last longer or run faster. According to the FDA, on the other hand, "energy" means calories, so sports bars are legally allowed to tout their energy (calorie)-promoting qualities. Athletes, however, don't benefit immediately from extra calories unless they're doing long-term (an hour or more) aerobic activities. If you want the extra calories, for whatever reason, you can get them from a sports bar — or from a bagel, a banana, or dried fruit. Sports bars are expensive, but they're also compact and don't get bruised or go stale in a few days. They can also be thrown into a gym bag and taken to tournaments, so they're great travel food — but not necessarily better than real food.

The Nutrition Box Score

- Aim for balance, moderation, and variety in the types of food your child eats.
- Try different foods and recipes with your kids.
- Hydration (water intake) is important before, during, and after activity.

Performance-Enhancing Drugs and Nutritional Supplements

Key Terms

Anabolic steroids. Synthetically produced testosterone derivatives that can be taken orally or injected into muscle and will increase baseline strength by increasing the anabolic (muscle-building) effects of testosterone. Can also predispose users to increased risk of liver cancer and other medical problems.

Androstenedione. Nutritional supplement touted by manufacturers as a "safe" alternative to anabolic steroids. This compound is not safe, has not been cleared by the FDA, and can cause premature puberty in kids and teens.

Creatine. Nutritional supplement taken by athletes to improve strength. Not recommended for children and adolescents due to absence of testing in this age group.

Diuretic. Drug causing rapid weight reduction through loss of water. Prescribed for patients with heart disease, it has also been abused by wrestlers to rapidly reduce weight.

Ergogenic substances. Also called performance-enhancing drugs, these are chemical compounds used by athletes to improve sports performance.

Nutritional supplements. A broad category of substances — none of which has ever been tested by the FDA (Food and Drug Administration) — that athletes (and nonathletes) take to improve performance. None of these compounds has been tested in children or teens, and the long-term safety is not known. Products include creatine, androstenedione, HMB, and ma juang.

Last year, the mother of a high school football star, Ed, called with serious concerns. "Dr. Metzl, last week Eddie was awarded a Division One football scholarship."

"That's great," I said. I had seen Ed for a shoulder injury the year before, and he had been hoping to play college football.

"His new coach called yesterday. He wants Eddie to start taking nutritional supplements to improve his strength."

I told the mother to have Ed see me in my office by next week. What I told him is what I am going to tell you: Performance-enhancing drugs — and this includes nutritional supplements — are bad news for athletes.

The broad term *ergogenic aid* means a drug taken to chemically improve performance (as opposed to improvement resulting from effort such as exercise or practice). *Ergogenic* comes from the Greek word meaning "to make work." Ergogenic aids build muscle, increase endurance, or change weight without the athlete's doing the work himself through training. That's one reason they're different from improved equipment (e.g., the swimmer's torpedo suit, the pole vaulter's aluminum pole), which are part of the game, available to all competitors, used openly, and cause no unhealthy side effects. Ergogenic aids include banned agents such as steroids, as well as so-called natural performance-enhancing agents such as creatine. These substances are a multimillion-dollar business, and their manufacturers have a financial interest in getting your kids to start using the products when they are young. Multiple studies have shown that people who start using a product as kids or teens (a brand of toothpaste or deodorant, for example) are more likely to use that product as adults. Even when companies know their products might be harmful, the profit motive of getting kids and teens to start using them often outweighs morality. One obvious example is cigarette companies, who used attractive icons like Joe Camel to encourage teens to start smoking and thus to buy cigarettes for their entire lives.

In some circles, the Sydney Summer Olympics of 2000 were known as the "Drug Olympics": eight athletes were caught using illegal drugs, and more than two hundred withdrew from competition when more stringent drug tests were announced just before the start of the games. Unfortunately, drugs are associated not only with Olympic athletes, but with all athletes, even those in high school and junior high.

As kids get older, they want to win. By the time athletes hit high school, and for boys in particular, in the words of Vince Lombardi, winning isn't everything, it's the only thing. As the focus turns more toward winning, and as the rewards — social, and in some cases, financial — for successful athletes become more significant, some kids and teens will adopt any method that can potentially improve their sports performance. One of the most popular, and also dangerous, routes is performance-enhancing drugs.

One widely quoted study on the 1998 U.S. Winter Olympics team asked athletes: "If you could take a performance-enhancing drug and not get caught, would you?" Over 90 percent answered yes. This same group was then asked, "If you could take the same undetectable substance, win every competition for five years, and then die, would you?" Over 50 percent said yes! When winning becomes the only focus, reason and perspective can take a back seat.

Parents should be aware that by the time their child is playing junior high school sports, other kids on the team are probably taking ergogenic substances that are banned and/or untested for long-term effects on adolescents. At the high school level, several studies have looked at user rates of anabolic steroids, among the most dangerous types of ergogenic aids. Most studies report 8 to 10 percent user rates of anabolic steroids in high school boys, and a recent study indicated that girls are beginning to take anabolic steroids as well. Even more shocking, a survey-study of junior high students found that 2 to 3 percent of junior high students reported taking anabolic steroids.

Take the time to understand ergogenic aids so you can discuss them with your child. We learned in the 1980s that the Nancy Reagan "Just say no" approach to drugs didn't work — the number of teens with drug problems increased rather than decreased. In order to tell your kids they shouldn't take ergogenic aids, you need to be able to explain *why* they shouldn't. The following table lists the common classes of ergogenic aids we see in high school.

Substance	Ergogenic Effect	Side Effects
Anabolic steroids (nandrolone, Dianabol) — used for football, strength sports.	Available in oral and injectable forms; can increase muscle strength by increasing testosterone level.	Premature puberty (boys). Development of facial hair (girls). Increased risk of hepatic (liver) cancer.
Diuretics (Lasix) — used for wrestling, swimming, sports in which weight is a handicap.	Rapid weight loss.	Can cause electrolyte abnormalities leading to cardiac arrhythmia.
Androstenedione (Andro) — used for strength sports.	Increases testosterone level, which increases muscle strength.	Same as for anabolic steroids.
Creatine	Increases muscle creatine, which can increase muscle strength in some adults in conjunction with lifting weights.	Water retention, possible increased risk of kidney failure.

All ergogenic aids are not the same. Some are clearly dangerous, such as anabolic steroids and diuretics, while some are billed as natural supplements, such as androstenedione and creatine. We know more about chemically manufactured substances such as anabolic steroids and diuretics because they have been better studied. In contrast, despite the potential dangers of nutritional or "natural" supplements, these compounds have not been researched by the Food and Drug Administration (FDA), and their long-term effects are not known. In addition, there is *no* government oversight whatsoever of the composition of supplements. When penicillin is manufactured, for example, an FDA supervision procedure ensures that what is written on the bottle's label and what is in the drug are identical. Because they are not regulated, the contents of a nutritional supplement bottle may be quite different from what is listed on its label.

Many athletes take literally hundreds of compounds to improve sports performance, so rather than list them all, I list the most important groups and describe how they work.

Anabolic Steroids

These are probably the most dangerous ergogenic aids that kids and teens can take, and also among the most common. Kids sometimes get them through high school teammates and sometimes through the sports black market. Steroid use tends to occur in clusters of kids rather than in isolated cases.

In "The Use of Anabolic-Androgenic Steroids in Sports" the American College of Sports Medicine states, "The use of anabolic-androgenic steroids by athletes is contrary to the rules and ethical principles of athletic competition as set forth by many of the sports governing bodies. The American College of Sports Medicine supports these ethical principles and deplores the use of anabolic-androgenic steroids by athletes."

Anabolic steroids are testosterone derivatives, meaning they come from the same chemical root as testosterone. These substances, first invented in the 1960s, were actually synthesized by scientists from testosterone, the male sex hormone. Anabolic steroids were designed to enhance the muscle-building function of testosterone while limiting the development of secondary sexual characteristics. Although thousands of scientists have tried to isolate the muscle-building effects, even the most high-end anabolic steroids still cause some degree of secondary sexual characteristic development, though less than if the athlete were taking straight testosterone. They are available in injectable and oral forms.

Taking testosterone results not only in getting stronger, but also in developing all the male secondary sexual characteristics such as facial hair, acne, and deepening voice. These changes can occur not just in males who take the drug but in females as well. In boys, it's important not to mistake normal behavioral or physical changes for evidence of anabolic steroid use. The naturally increased testosterone levels in the adolescent male typically result in increased strength, acne, and emotional instability (impulsive behaviors, hyperactivity, inability to sit still, aggression, even rage). However, if these changes seem way out of proportion to normal, or if your kid is getting in fights all the time, it's important to think about anabolic steroids as the cause.

Signs of Anabolic Steroid Use

It's tough to know for sure, but the cardinal signs to watch out for include

- Rapid change in body build (doctors call this *habitus*) compared to peers, with muscle being put on much more quickly than previously and compared to peers ("Jim is much stronger than he used to be").
- Psychological symptoms: rage, temper, aggressiveness, getting into fights.
- Rapid onset of acne.

What to Do If You Suspect Anabolic Steroid Use

1. **Discuss steroid use with your child.** The first and most important thing is to talk to your kid. Both parents should be involved. Take your child to a neutral site, away from home and distractions such as siblings, and discuss your concerns honestly and openly. Don't go behind his back!

2. **Get professional help.** Even if your child says, "I won't do this anymore, I promise," he probably will. As with the Olympians in the study cited above, when winning becomes the only focus, thinking turns cloudy. Given that other kids are likely to be taking performance-enhancing drugs, the best thing to do is to seek help outside the school. Start with your pediatrician. A local adolescent-medicine doctor (a pediatrician who specializes in adolescent-health issues) would also be an important resource.

3. **Use thoughtful discouragement.** If kids are taking anabolic steroids, they are almost certainly taking them to improve their sports performance. Parents and coaches need to understand that

these substances work: athletes actually do get stronger and faster with anabolic steroids. You must acknowledge these benefits before discouraging use or you will lose credibility with your child. You must also point out, however, that the downside of anabolic steroids outweighs the good. Using these substances increases the risk of liver cancer, heart disease, stroke, and infertility, and in kids who haven't started puberty, they decrease adult size.

4. **Discuss ergogenic aids with other parents**. If you see a rat in your garbage one morning, the odds are great that many other rats are in the vicinity. The same is true of steroid users. If one athlete is caught taking steroids, chances are many others on the team are doing the same thing. For parents, it's important not to bury your head in the sand and pretend that it couldn't be happening with your child. If others on the team are doing this, your child has at least thought about it too.

Anabolic Steroid Use in Girls

Although anabolic steroid use is primarily a male issue, increasing numbers of female athletes are taking these substances. Why? Because females, who normally secrete very low levels of testosterone, can gain even more dramatic results from anabolic steroid use than males can. This is because testosterone stimulates muscle building; testosterone is the primary reason that boys become so much stronger than girls during puberty. When females take anabolic steroids, their muscles greatly increase in strength, but they also develop male secondary sexual characteristics, such as acne, facial hair, and deepening voice. These are the same symptoms of steroid use in boys, but should be more evident with girls because any slight increase in their low levels of testosterone leads to abnormal physical changes. As the financial rewards for athletic success continue to grow for females, the push to win at all costs is increasingly becoming part of the women's and girls' sports world. In the future, we will probably see more anabolic steroid use in female athletes, so it's important for parents to recognize the symptoms of use in girls.

Diuretics

Diuretics are drugs used to increase the volume of urine, which decreases extra water weight. They are prescribed for patients who have too much fluid in their tissues, for example as the result of a weakened heart.

In 1999, four young wrestlers died within a two-month period — three in college and one in high school — all from diuretic use. Wrestlers, who compete in a weight category, often find themselves with only a day to lose four or five pounds in order to "make weight." No one knows the prevalence of diuretic use among athletes, but it almost certainly goes on much more than we can document. We only hear about the problems once they become catastrophic.

Diuretics are dangerous because they alter the ratio of ions in the body, particularly sodium and potassium, thereby changing the water distribution in cells. For this reason, patients who take diuretics are monitored closely by their physician, and blood tests are routinely conducted to check the ion ratio. College and Olympic athletes who take diuretics can be banned from competition for years, and aside from the moral issue of cheating, there is no mechanism to ensure safe ion ratios. Taking diuretics without medical supervision can result in the sodium level dropping too low or the potassium level getting too high. When either of these occurs, there is a significant risk of heart arrhythmia, a change in how the heart beats. All four of the 1999 wrestling deaths were due to arrhythmia.

A wrestler who loses weight rapidly to make a particular weight class is also likely to lose the match. A study of wrestlers who dropped pounds quickly (about eight pounds, or 4.5 percent of their body weight) found that they performed 3.5 percent worse on a six-minute arm crank test intended to simulate a wrestling competition. The reason is loss of muscle glycogen and dehydration. In sum: Diuretics can be deadly and don't help you win.

Signs of Diuretic Use

It can be very difficult to detect whether an athlete is taking diuretics, but important clues can help parents investigate these issues further. These include:

- Are other kids on the team taking diuretics?
- Has your child undergone rapid weight loss, out of proportion to other teammates? Whereas dancers might get skinnier over a period of months, athletes taking diuretics get thin over a period of days. They tend to look haggard, with dry eyes and tightly drawn cheeks, because all of the water is pulled right out of the tissues.
- Does your child urinate frequently? Someone taking diuretics urinates "all the time." If your child is trying to "make weight" and starts urinating more than six or seven times a day, it's probably a good idea to ask whether he is taking diuretics.

Nutritional Supplements

Promoted as "safer and natural" alternatives to drugs such as anabolic steroids, nutritional supplements or "natural compounds" in pill or powder form are being marketed, bought, and sold at an amazing rate over the Internet and in health-food stores. Nutritional supplements are a multimillion-dollar-a-year industry, and many of them are being directed toward teenagers who want "the right look." Popular nutritional supplements include androstenedione, creatine, and other health-food products marketed under names such as "rip fuel" and "instant strength."

Parents need to know that no nutritional supplements have ever been tested on teens or kids, and the safety — short-term as well as long-term — of these products is completely unknown. In 1993, the FDA removed nutritional supplements from its jurisdiction, thereby opening a Pandora's box. Anyone — including children and teenagers — can walk into a health-food store and buy these products. The issue that concerns medical professionals is that without FDA regulation, there is no control over what is actually in these pills and powders known as "nutritional supplements." Besides the possibility of their causing detrimental health effects, these products may create problems for unsuspecting athletes when they undergo drug tests. Many college and Olympic athletes using these supplements have tested positive for banned substances, such as anabolic steroids. Since nutritional supplements are not regulated, a product labeled as a muscle-building protein powder with amino acids might actually contain anabolic steroids as well.

A study published in the *New England Journal of Medicine* found that people taking ma juang, a nutritional supplement designed to increase energy, were about 20 to 25 times more likely than a control group to suffer strokes. Because it is a nutritional supplement, it was never tested by the FDA. Thinking it was healthy and safe, people took it and died (over a three-year period, thirty-two people died in California alone). Ma juang used to be found in almost every health-food store across the country, but after the study, it was pulled from the shelves.

Androstenedione (Andro)

Androstenedione is a nutritional supplement designed to increase strength by increasing the amount of testosterone in the body. Testosterone is created in a series of stages, called a pathway. Androstenedione is the last step on the pathway to testosterone and is known as a steroid precursor. In 1998, Mark McGwire of the St. Louis Cardinals made andro famous when he took it and broke the single-season home run record. Some questioned whether his prowess came from his own hard work, or from the effects of andro.

To answer this question, Major League Baseball commissioned Harvard Medical School to assess the effect of andro on testosterone levels. The study found that if taken in moderate to high doses, andro does increase testosterone. For a physically mature athlete like McGwire, this means more testosterone is available to make muscle. But for kids and teens, the effects are very different.

As noted in Chapter 5, rising testosterone levels signal the start of puberty in boys. If boys take andro, the extra testosterone starts puberty too early (called *premature puberty*). In addition, taking andro can make the testicles shrink because the body's response to the higher levels of testosterone in the blood is to have the testicles stop producing more of it. The end result is that since they start growing too early, boys can end up being shorter and having smaller testicles than they would normally — not the desired effect. In girls, andro can cause facial hair growth and acne.

However, andro is a nutritional supplement that is legally and easily available, so kids and teens can and do take it. It's important to explain how it can affect them, and if necessary, seek the help of your pediatrician. Many kids, teens, and even some parents think that andro is "natural," so it must be safe. Nothing is further from the truth. Remember, arsenic and cocaine are also natural substances.

Creatine

Creatine, another "natural supplement," is increasingly being used by teens and kids to enhance their athletic performance. Creatine is an amino acid produced in the body by the kidneys and pancreas and is also ingested in meats and fish. The total amount that most humans need is about 2 grams a day, half of which comes from the body and half from food. We need creatine to function well: it facilitates muscle contraction. The manufacturers of creatine supplements, however, would have us believe that creatine increases strength, and that if a little creatine is good, then more is better.

In a 1999 study in the Northeast, we asked athletes in grades six through twelve whether they were taking creatine. We found that more than 7 percent of respondents answered yes. There were male and female users in every grade, although more boys used it than girls. Among twelfth graders, the rate was a shocking 44 percent of all athletes.

The questions about creatine are: (1) Does it increase strength? (2) Is it safe? and (3) Should my kids take it? In short: (1) We are not sure whether creatine works. Some athletes seem to be able to lift more weight or hit harder by taking it, but most are not. (2) Three cases of permanent kidney failure attributed to creatine use have been reported, and the long-term effects have never been studied. (3) Absolutely not. We have no idea what the long-term effects of creatine might be. It is worth remembering that when cigarettes first came out, they were widely promoted as a method of improving vitality.

What to do if you suspect your child is taking creatine? The familiar refrain here is that performance-enhancing drug use travels in groups. If one kid on the football team is taking creatine, certainly others are too. Be sure to discuss with kids and teens that we don't know what this substance does and that we're not even sure it works. They might well be wasting money on something we don't know enough about; worse, they might be damaging their health and development over the long run.

It's also a good idea to have a doctor discuss these drugs at a team meeting with the coach and players. Because the coach spends so much more time with the athletes than other adults do, giving him information about the long-term implications as well as symptoms can be very helpful.

The Other Supplements: Health Food Powders and Vitamins

Literally thousands of products, powders, and mixes are listed on the Internet and at nutrition stores as performance-enhancing. "Protein powder," "Vita-mix," "Energy Boost" are only a few of these products. They may not be pills, but that doesn't make them safe. If your child or teen wants to take one of these, and you are having a tough time discouraging her, please take the time to consult a nutritionist, preferably one specializing in sports nutrition. You can find a nutritionist through your pediatrician, or even through a local gym, coach, or athletic director. Be sure your nutritionist is an R.D. (Registered Dietician), which certifies that he or she has completed a specific school program that ensures a basic level of knowledge. Dieticians who have pursued extra training in sports nutrition are the most qualified to answer questions about performance-enhancing drugs, nutritional supplements, and health-food powders and vitamins. None of these has been tested in kids, and no young athlete should take any without speaking to a doctor or sports nutritionist.

The Final Argument

While it is true that ergogenic aids can improve performance, the reasons not to use them are

- These substances haven't been tested on adolescents for long-term effects on health and development.
- The substances that have been tested on adults result in deleterious effects on long-term and sometimes short-term health; some are fatal.
- There is no personal satisfaction or growth from winning by cheating — by having a chemical do the work instead of your own effort. The primary reason to play sports should be the personal satisfaction of doing the best you can through your own work.

Whenever you're trying to dissuade kids from doing something that's bad for them, don't be merely negative. It's important to give them an alternative, constructive route to their goals. Get the kids to the gym and the practice field. Have them start lifting weights, doing strength training. Encourage preseason conditioning, an established and much more effective way of improving strength, fitness, endurance, and performance. Furthermore, the athlete is doing the work that is the point of sports, instead of resorting to the quick fix of drugs.

The Nutritional Supplements and Drugs Box Score

- Recognize use patterns.
- Discuss ergogenic aids openly and honestly with your children.
- Use thoughtful discouragement after understanding the issues yourself.
- Develop other avenues for improving performance.

Chapter 7

Preparing for the Sports Season

PRESEASON CONDITIONING AND TRAINING

Getting in shape before the season starts improves athletic performance and helps reduce injuries.

essica, a twelve-year-old basketball player, wants to make her school team. Ryan, a nine-year-old football player, wants to play with older kids. Amy, an eight-year-old figure skater, wants to start jumping. Julianne, a sixteen-year-old swimmer, wants to make the varsity team. And Keith, a fourteen-year-old pitcher, wants to make the summer league baseball team.

What do these young athletes have in common? The differences are more apparent than their similarities: different ages, different genders, different sports. The similarity is that each one can benefit from effective preseason conditioning: getting into shape before the first practice. For athletes of any age, but particularly for young athletes, this can make a tremendous difference in performance — jumping higher, running or swimming faster, throwing harder.

When team practice starts, especially for the fall sports season, two types of young athletes generally show up: those who have spent the summer lounging by the pool, playing video games, and eating

Key Terms

Avulsion fracture. A fracture in which a tendon pulls off a piece of bone, usually at the site of a cartilage growth plate.

Cardiovascular conditioning. "Heart and lung" conditioning. Getting "in shape" for the season means exercising your heart and lungs to increase their capacity. Like other muscles, these need to get in shape as well.

Exercise-induced asthma (EIA). Shortness of breath and wheezing during and just after intense physical activity. It is not the same as asthma (the actual medical term for EIA is *exercise-induced bronchospasm*), and it is present in 95 percent of asthmatics and roughly 15 to 20 percent of the nonasthmatic population.

Power lifting. Maximum weight lifting, trying to "max out" for two or three repetitions. It is not safe for kids or teens, because of the potential for growth plate injury.

Preseason conditioning. Getting in shape for the sports season, starting about six weeks before practice begins. Conditioning should address both cardiovascular and muscular conditioning.

Strength training. Repetitive weight lifting using light weights and many repetitions to build strength. Though safe for kids and teens, it needs to be supervised by adults.

hamburgers, and those who have taken off-season conditioning seriously. The second group is more likely to improve once practice begins because they can concentrate on skills instead of on getting into shape. With increased muscular strength, the trained group is less likely to be injured and more apt to have a favorable sports experience.

Regardless of the age and the chosen sport of your young athlete — whether a seven-year-old soccer player, a thirteen-year-old field hockey star, or a seventeen-year-old swimmer — preseason conditioning will help her perform better on the field, and also help keep her out of my office. Encourage your kids to start preseason conditioning (and start cutting down on video games and junk food) about six weeks before the opening of the sports season. I even know some families in which the parents and kids do these programs together.

Preseason conditioning can be divided into two types: *cardiovascular*, designed to enhance the heart and lungs, and *muscular*, designed to increase muscle strength and bone density. Both types are important, and if properly done, can improve performance and safety.

Cardiovascular Conditioning

Cardiovascular conditioning can take any form and is best accomplished by letting kids be kids. The key is to encourage them to develop a consistent activity pattern, usually four to five days of vigorous exercise a week. Unlike strength training, which is often sport-specific (for example, the muscles a figure skater needs to strengthen to improve jumping ability are very different from those a pitcher develops to throw a baseball), cardiovascular conditioning is generalized. The heart and lungs don't care what kind of activity someone is doing, they just care that they are being properly exercised. When figure skaters play basketball or football players swim, they not only increase their cardiovascular fitness and work different muscles, they also develop different skill sets, and it's fun, too.

Cardiovascular Conditioning and Asthma

Cardiovascular conditioning is important for all young athletes, but it is especially important for those with asthma or exercise-induced asthma (EIA). Asthma is the most common medical condition in kids and teens, affecting about 3 to 5 percent of this age group.

> ## Keys to Increasing Cardiovascular Fitness
> - Start a cardiovascular conditioning program five to six weeks before the sports season begins. If your child is at summer camp, encourage her to get on a running program there before she returns home.
> - Exercise 30 to 40 minutes, four to five times a week.
> - Keep it fun. Any activity your child enjoys that keeps the heart rate up — tennis, swimming, soccer, basketball — will improve cardiovascular fitness.

When kids have asthma attacks, they become short of breath and start wheezing. These episodes can happen at any time and can be terrifying for kids, parents, and coaches. Another group of kids and teens have exercise-induced asthma; they have problems with shortness of breath and wheezing *only* when playing sports. They are not asthmatics (the actual medical term is *exercise-induced bronchospasm*, not asthma), and they usually have never had an asthma "attack." The only time shortness of breath is a problem is during intense physical activity. EIA is much more common than asthma, estimated to affect about 12 to 14 percent of the general population. African Americans are at highest risk, for reasons we don't understand.

As athletes improve their cardiovascular fitness, their lungs are more able to tolerate exercise, and they breathe easier during and after sports. If you have an asthmatic or EIA athlete at home, you have probably noticed that she uses her inhaler (asthma medicine) much less frequently as the sports season progresses. By being sure she is in top cardiovascular shape before the sports season starts, you can make the beginning of the season much more pleasant for everyone.

Summer Fitness Routine

This is a program given by a soccer coach to his team. Your child can take this as a starting point to discuss with her own coach. Most good coaches will prepare something similar for their players.

Remember, the key to this program's success is to do it consistently. Shoot for 30–45 minutes a day for five days. Take the weekend off from the program for either matches or to relax. Remember to stretch before and after workouts as well.

1. For treadmill:
   - 30 minutes — ¾ pace for 4 minutes, full speed for 2 minutes, and then back to ¾ pace.
   - After 30 minutes of interval running, 15 minutes at a slower pace to build stamina.

Ab workout: crunches and leg lifts (3 sets of 20). Don't overwork the abs; you won't get results.

2. If a field is accessible:
   - 30 minutes—jog length, sprint width.
     When you jog, the pace is only a bit faster than a walk.
     When you sprint, go full sprint.
     Really feel the drastic change in pace from jog to sprint.
   - After 15, 20 yds. high-knees sprints.

Ab workout: same as above.

Do this workout consistently for a month, and you will feel the difference.

Muscular Conditioning: Strength Training

Strength training increases muscle power, improves bone density, and is generally helpful for all athletes. Increasingly, the medical community is recognizing the importance of strength training for athletes of all ages. In my practice, I have patients as young as eight and as old as eighty on strength-training programs.

Strength Training versus Power Lifting

When I give talks to parent groups and come to the part on strength training, I often get quizzical looks. "Julia is only nine," parents say, "and I don't want her to look like Arnold Schwarzenegger." It's important to distinguish between strength training and weight training. Strength training is repetitive lifting of light weights, designed to increase baseline strength by developing more muscle fiber. Power lifting is heavy lifting designed to maximize muscle bulk.

Strength training is safe for kids; power lifting is not. The bones of children and teens end in open growth plates made of cartilage, and power lifting is potentially dangerous to growth plates. If a child or teen tries to apply a maximum force across the growth plate, he can pull off the end of the bone; this is called an *avulsion fracture*. John, an eleven-year-old, became my patient when he tried to impress his older brother with his weight-lifting ability. Attempting a biceps curl with too much weight, he actually pulled off part of the growth plate at the end of his arm, an avulsion fracture, and needed surgery to repair it.

How Does Strength Training Work in Kids?

Strength-training programs employ multiple repetitions of a combination of resistance activities (weights, push-ups, and so on) to increase baseline strength, which is essential to all sports. I encourage strength-training programs for all children and teens who are serious about their sport. It makes them play better, prevents injury, and is an important method of preparation. But kids need to know that the results of a strength-training program aren't visible. The muscles don't get bigger, they get stronger. Kids, even as young as eight or nine, can increase their strength by 40 to 50 percent over a six-week period.

When adult males lift weights, their muscles get bigger through a process called *muscle hypertrophy*, which is largely caused by normally circulating testosterone levels. The higher the testosterone level, the more the muscle cells respond to training by thickening. An eleven-year-old boy's testosterone levels are low, so when he is involved in a weight-lifting program, his muscles don't get bigger. When puberty starts, however, the testosterone levels increase, and the same weight-lifting program will make that athlete's muscles hypertrophy. (The low level of testosterone in adult females is why they do not bulk up the way males do.) Strength training in kids does not work through muscle hypertrophy, but through increased recruitment of muscle fibers. Unlike adults, who get stronger when the muscle cells get bigger, kids get stronger when more of their muscle is called to action. The bodies of most kids and teens use only 50 to 60 percent of the capacity of the muscles involved in a given activity. When a muscle is strength-trained, more of it is utilized.

Boys, even when young, want strong, articulated muscles and are often discouraged when their strength-training program doesn't produce these visible results. Girls, on the other hand, generally don't want bigger muscles. It's important to tell both boys and girls that the changes in the muscle from strength training happen inside and are nearly invisible. Rather than see the results, they will feel them. Neither boys nor girls will look like Arnold, but they'll both get stronger.

A final point here about anabolic steroids: Athletes who take them are raising their level of testosterone. Instead of developing strength through increased muscle fiber recruitment, young athletes taking steroids will develop enlarged muscles through hypertrophy, which can put too much stress on the unfinished growth plates. That is, the muscles become too strong for the level of skeletal development, and the bones aren't ready for that amount of force. So aside from long-term health risks such as the increased likelihood of

developing cancer, steroid use by children can also result in significant and potentially long-term growth-plate injuries.

Starting a Strength-Training Program at Home

Now that you're convinced that strength training is a good idea for
your young athlete, how do you start? Actually, your child would
probably benefit most by joining her teammates in an off-season
program at school or a fitness center, run by professionals with all
the proper equipment. But if this is not feasible for practical or financial reasons, a home-based strength-training program is a very
acceptable alternative, with the added potential benefit of family
togetherness. (Kids who go away to camp can also use the program
described below, always provided they are supervised by a responsible adult.) The key is to make your program easy, accessible, and
fun. Incorporate it into your child's weekly routine; maybe join in
yourself. As kids grow and realize their parents aren't "cool," finding
meaningful activities to share with them becomes more difficult.
Developing a strength-training program with your kids or teens will
not only help their sports performance, it can also be a great way for
parents and kids to spend quality time together.

> The Keys to an Effective Strength-Training Program
> - Have kids start five to six weeks before the sports season, two or
>   three times a week.
> - Parents must supervise (essential for kids under sixteen years of
>   age who lift weights).
> - Be organized (keep progress charts on the wall and fill them in
>   together; make it part of the daily schedule).
> - Make it fun.

This program should be repeated three times a week, starting
about five or six weeks before the sports season begins. I want to
emphasize that it requires adult supervision at all times. If your child

starts to complain of pain, it's important to stop and discuss the program with a pediatrician or sports medicine physician.

To use this home-based strengthening program you will need:

- two 3-pound dumbbells
- two 5-pound dumbbells
- one 5-pound ankle weight
- one 10-pound ankle weight
- one 15-pound ankle weight
- At least one supportive supervising parent for athletes under sixteen

Almost all the exercises are done in three sets of 15 repetitions each. The third set of 15 should be a little taxing but not painful. Most important: Let your young athlete decide when the weight is sufficient. Remember that we are activating more muscle fibers here, not going after muscle hypertrophy. So even if it doesn't hurt, it's working!

Leg Strengthening
RUNNING-BASED AND JUMPING-BASED SPORTS

Leg strength is important for all sports, but especially for running-based and jumping sports such as basketball, soccer, lacrosse, figure skating, field hockey, and football. Baseball pitchers also need to focus on leg strengthening to help push off when throwing.

The two major muscle groups of the legs that respond to strength training are the quadriceps (quads) and hamstrings. The quads make up the front of the thigh, the hamstrings the back of the thigh. It's very important to try to create an equal balance between quadriceps and hamstring strength, especially in female athletes. Imbalance between quad and hamstring strength is posited as a major reason that female athletes are much more likely to tear their ACL (anterior cruciate ligament) than males: when the front leg muscles are stronger than the back muscles and the knee is stressed, the thigh is pulled forward, thus tearing the ACL. The quads are naturally bigger and stronger muscles than the hamstrings, but the goal is to balance these muscle groups as much as possible.

These illustrations show two common methods of quad strengthening. Figure 3 shows how to use ankle weights to extend the leg
against the resistance of gravity. Three sets of 15 repetitions on each
leg are sufficient. Rest for 30 seconds between sets. The athlete
should be able to do all three sets of 15, but choose a weight that
makes the muscle feel tired at the end of the third set of 15.

Figure 3.
Quadriceps-muscle strengthening with leg
extension and ankle weights.

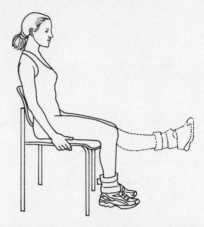

Figure 4 shows another method of quad strengthening: squats
while holding dumbbells. Repeat for three sets of 15 for each leg,
again using enough weight to make the muscle feel tired at the end
of the third set. After each set of 15, switch legs so the front leg
changes.

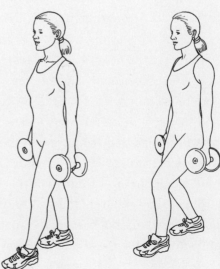

Figure 4.
Alternative quadriceps-muscle
strengthening with dumbbells.

Hamstring Strengthening

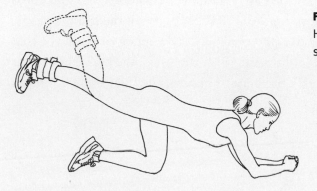

Figure 5.
Hamstring
strengthening.

Hamstring strengthening is the only proven prevention strategy for ACL injuries, so all athletes, but especially female athletes, need to engage in hamstring-strengthening exercises for six weeks before the start of sports season (and it's probably a good idea to do these year round). At-risk female athletes include participants in field sports such as soccer, field hockey, and lacrosse. Female basketball players run three to four times the risk of tearing their ACL as their male peers.

Figure 5 shows the ankle-weight method of hamstring strengthening. Allow the weight to come up and down slowly. Each leg should do three sets of 15 repetitions, and again, the muscle should be fatigued by the end of the third repetition.

Core Strengthening: The Abdominal and Lower Back Muscles
ALL SPORTS, ALL AGES, BUT ESPECIALLY SOCCER, FOOTBALL, BALLET

The key to a happy body is a strong core. These exercises will benefit any athlete, regardless of age or sport. Many of my patients are able to exercise regularly into their seventies, eighties, and even nineties because they have strong cores.

The *core* is the term doctors use to refer to the combined strength of the abdominal muscles ("abs") and the low-back muscles. Much like the quad and hamstring muscles in the leg, the abs and low-back muscles are the force groups that flank the lower back. When these muscles are strong, the spine is straight and back pain is less common. When these muscles are weak, the person often has bad posture, but more important, the vertebrae (bones of the spine) and the discs (cartilage between the vertebrae) take much of the force that stronger muscles would absorb. Over the years, the constant pounding can result in a bad back and significantly affect the individual's quality of life.

Abdominal Strengthening

Figure 6.
Dual-motion
abdominal muscle
strengthening.

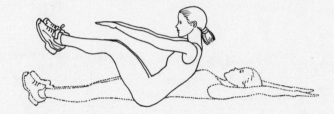

The abs can be strengthened in many ways. I have found the most effective method to be the combined motion of arms and legs, illustrated in Figure 6. Lie flat on your back and then slowly bring the extended arms and bent legs together. When they overlap, lie back down slowly. This should be done for three sets of 15 repetitions. Parents, do this with your kids!

Some kids, especially those under ten, find the dual-action method of abdominal strengthening too difficult. In this case, try crunches instead. These are also done in three sets of 15 repetitions, and are easier to master. See Figure 7.

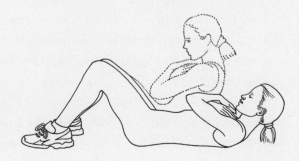

Figure 7.
Abdominal crunches for
muscle strengthening.

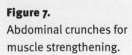

Low-Back Strengthening

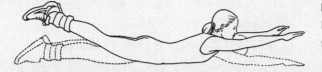

Figure 8.
Low-back
strengthening.

Again, there are many ways to achieve good low-back strength, but the best is the "Superman" technique, illustrated in Figure 8. The athlete lies flat, face down, and then extends both legs and arms, like Superman flying. Do this slowly and hold at the top for a few seconds. Three sets of 15 repetitions are usually sufficient.

Shoulder Strengthening
ESPECIALLY FOR OVERHEAD SPORTS: SWIMMING, TENNIS, BASEBALL, PITCHING IN BASEBALL, QUARTERBACKING IN FOOTBALL

The shoulder-strengthening exercises are important for all overhead athletes, including tennis players and swimmers, as well as throwing athletes such as baseball players and football quarterbacks. The shoulder is a part of the body where an ounce of prevention is worth about 25 pounds of cure. It is far, far better to spend a few minutes a week strengthening the rotator cuff muscles in the shoulder during the preseason than to waste weeks and sometimes months of a season trying to make these muscles stronger once they are sore and injured (see Chapter 9 on common upper-body injuries). Encourage your children to take the long-term view!

The rotator cuff, located inside the shoulder, consists of four small muscles that are responsible for making the shoulder work properly during overhead activities. Every time a tennis ball is served, every time a baseball is thrown, every time a freestyle stroke is made, the rotator cuff muscles are working hard, keeping the shoulder properly aligned. These muscles are dependent on each other, so equal strength between them is needed to keep the shoulder in a centered position. It's tricky to recognize weakness in the rotator cuff before actual injury. But pay attention to pain in the shoulder during or after overhead activities and see a doctor if such pain becomes a regular occurrence. Although most people don't walk around thanking their rotator cuff, I guarantee you will know it's there if it isn't strong enough!

The key to rotator cuff strengthening is making the muscles fit enough to stand up to the load of overhead sports. The swimmer who had shoulder pain last year from swimming increasing distances can probably prevent a recurrence by strengthening the rotator cuff muscles. The same is true of baseball and tennis players.

The three exercises shown in Figures 9, 10, and 11 — external rotation, internal rotation, and straight-arm extension — are designed to strengthen the rotator cuff muscles and need to be done together to ensure good muscle balance. Do these exercises with a dumbbell; 3 pounds is plenty for most kids and teens (kids might even prefer a soup can instead of a weight).

External Rotation

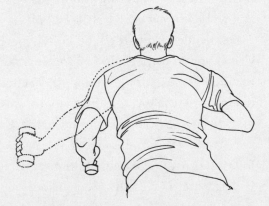

Figure 9.
External-rotation strengthening.

External-rotation strengthening is accomplished by lying on the stomach over a bench or sofa, with the arm tucked in at 90 degrees. Figure 9 shows the proper technique for external rotation, strengthening the rotator cuff muscles on the back of the shoulder. Let the arm face downward, and then slowly bring the arm to a horizontal position, then back down to a vertical (or neutral) position, where there is no stress on the shoulder. Three sets of 15 repetitions for each arm are usually sufficient.

Internal Rotation

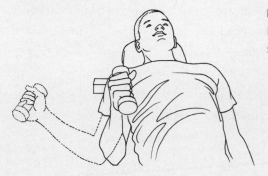

Figure 10.
Internal-rotation
strengthening.

Figure 10 shows the proper technique for internal rotation, strengthening the rotator cuff muscle group in the front of the shoulder. The athlete lies on his back, with the arm flat on the floor, elbow angled at 90 degrees. The arm is allowed to slowly rotate to the neutral position (sticking straight up), and then back to the horizontal 90-degree position. Three sets of 15 repetitions for each arm are sufficient, and don't be surprised if the internal-rotation strength is greater than the external-rotation strength. This is normal. Most people can tolerate about 5 pounds of weight with internal-rotation strengthening, as distinct from using 3 pounds for external rotation. There is no rule about weights here except to use what is comfortable.

Straight-Arm Extension

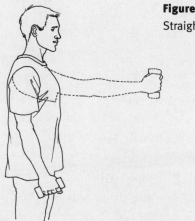

Figure 11.
Straight-arm extension.

The third set of exercises to strengthen the rotator cuff involves the upper part of the shoulder. Figure 11 shows the proper technique, holding a dumbbell and keeping the arm straight, lifting upward against gravity. Again, do three sets of 15 repetitions for each arm, and slowly, please.

Note: The easiest way to reach the desired three sets of each exercise is to do 15 reps of each one, then repeat all three exercises twice more.

Forearm Strengthening
BASEBALL, TENNIS

The forearm muscles are responsible for controlling the power exerted by the wrist, so strengthening these muscles during preseason is particularly important for baseball players to help with their throwing and batting. Forearm strengthening is often helpful for tennis players as well. Especially at the junior high and high school level, tennis players will notice that their groundstrokes are stronger.

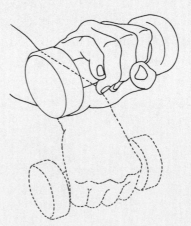

Figure 12.
Forearm strengthening.

Figure 12 shows a simple method of forearm strengthening using a dumbbell. For most children or teens, the 3-pound dumbbell provides sufficient resistance, but the 5- and even 7-pound weight can be used by older teens. In this exercise, the dumbbell is slowly raised against resistance in sets of 15 repetitions for each hand. It is easiest to let the wrist hang over the edge of a table, and then extend the wrist upward. This strengthens the forearm muscles, which helps prevent throwing-related elbow injuries as well as tennis elbow.

Chest Strengthening
ALL SPORTS, BUT PARTICULARLY FOOTBALL, BASKETBALL, WRESTLING

The chest muscles (pectorals, or "pecs") protect the front of the torso and help to generate force in high-contact sports, such as football and wrestling. Strengthening these muscles is very useful for most athletes; for example, basketball and soccer players with strong pecs are better able to muscle their opponents out of position or off the ball. Again, remember that we're not out to win the Arnold Schwarzenegger look-alike contest; strength, not size, is the key.

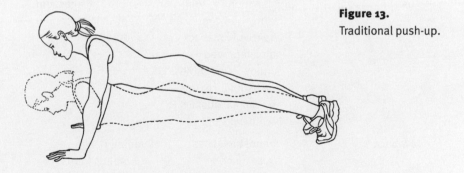

Figure 13.
Traditional push-up.

The key to good chest muscle strength is consistently doing sets of push-ups: three sets of 10 to 15, three times a week. I disapprove of differentiating between the "male" and "female" push-up because I think both genders are able to do the traditional push-up. This method, pictured in Figure 13, allows for maximum resistance against body weight and optimal strength improvement. Push-ups are portable, inexpensive, and a great habit for life.

The best way to ensure that your young athlete is following the optimal conditioning program is to ask the coach of the local high school team what type of sports-specific preseason conditioning program he uses, and try to implement a program like it for your

	Preseason Training	
Muscles	**Results of Strength Training**	**Sports It Benefits**
Quads	Faster running, higher jumping, stronger push-off when throwing. Short bursts of speed and jumping ability.	Running-based and jumping sports: basketball, soccer, lacrosse, figure skating, football; pitching in baseball.
Hamstrings	Reduced chance of ACL injuries. Better long-distance running ability.	Running-based sports: soccer, track, football, basketball.
Abs	Well-functioning, long-lasting body; reduced chance of low-back pain. Improved cardiovascular fitness due to ability to use abdominal muscles to breathe easier.	All sports, all ages, but especially soccer, football, dance.
Low back	Better posture. Less stress on bone structures in spine. Better running form, better jumping ability.	Running-based and jumping sports: basketball, soccer, lacrosse, figure skating, football.
Shoulder (rotator cuff)	Shoulder working properly with overhead activities, reduction of injuries.	Swimming, tennis, baseball, pitching in baseball, quarterbacking in football.
Forearm	More powerful wrist flexion and extension.	Baseball, tennis.
Chest	Protection of the front of the torso and generation of force in high-contact sports.	All sports, but especially football, basketball, wrestling.

athlete. Ideally (as mentioned above), he or one of his colleagues should run such a program. See if you can find a way to make that happen. (An added benefit is the camaraderie developed among team members, which contributes to wins in the season.) But a home-exercise program is certainly a worthy alternative to a school-based program.

The Internet is also a terrific source of information, and also a way to contact other parents and kids around the world who are engaged in similar sports. But use the Internet judiciously — it contains bad information as well as good. Verify anything you find there with your doctor.

> ## The Box Score
> - Preseason conditioning improves performance and prevents injury.
> - Preseason conditioning involves two types of fitness: cardiovascular (heart, lungs) and muscular (muscle strength and bone density).

Chapter 8

Overuse Injury

WHAT HAPPENS WHEN KIDS DO TOO MUCH

This chapter will help parents recognize when kids are doing too much, and what effects excess activity has on their bodies. It will explain some of the common overuse injuries.

Parents often ask me "Is my child doing too much?" In Chapter 4, I discussed this question in relation to general lifestyle issues, such as whether the child is becoming overly sports-oriented to the detriment of her overall development. But the question frequently comes up in the context of overuse injuries, such as a hockey player playing six days a week who hurts his back or a baseball player pitching five days a week who incurs elbow pain.

In children, as in adults, these injuries develop *over time with increased activity* because of repetitive stress on normal bone. They're a clear signal that an athlete is doing too much. The more active he is, the worse the injury becomes. These injuries are common in pounding sports such as running and soccer, but also in repetitive-loading sports such as dance and figure skating. When a patient complains of pain, I usually look at several issues, such as the type of sports the athlete is involved with, the type of injury he is developing, and the amount of time spent on the sport. Most kids can tolerate a lot of

Key Terms

Biomechanics. How someone is built as related to sports. The most common biomechanical problem is pronation, or "rolling in," of the feet, which predisposes an athlete to stress fractures in the feet, legs, and hips. Players can retrain muscles with faulty movement patterns to move efficiently and effectively.

Exercise-Induced Asthma (EIA). Shortness of breath and wheezing during and just after intense physical activity. It is not the same as asthma (the actual medical term for EIA is *exercise-induced bronchospasm*), and it is present in 95 percent of asthmatics and roughly 15 to 20 percent of the nonasthmatic population.

MRI (magnetic resonance imaging). A computer-generated image that uses a magnetic field to show the soft tissues (tendon, ligament, muscle, and cartilage) and their injuries.

Overuse Injury. Injury from doing "too much." Causes tissue breakdown. Athletes complain of pain that seems to worsen over time. Most overuse injuries are preventable with good preseason conditioning and proper biomechanics.

Stress Fracture. Overuse injury of the bone that results when too much stress is placed on the bone, causing the cortex (outside layer) to crack.

Stress Injury. Precursor of a stress fracture. The cortex is irritated but does not crack. Stress injury is easier to treat than stress fracture.

Tendinitis. Overuse injury of the tendon, such as Achilles tendinitis.

X-Rays. X-rays show bones, but not soft tissue such as tendon, ligament, muscle, and cartilage.

athletic activity, even as much as three hours a day. But there is such a thing as "too much," which is different for every child. Some kids will develop overuse injuries from moderate activity, while others never do, no matter what. In general, overuse injury is best treated by curing the injury and addressing the causative factors.

How do I know if my child or teen is doing too much?

When it comes to injuries, there is definitely such a thing as "too much." If a kid has missed more than 15 percent of the sports season with an overuse injury, I generally recommend that she see a sports medicine physician to determine if something can be done to help prevent a recurrence.

To help explain overuse injury, I'll describe both *tendinitis* and *stress fracture*. Both are common examples of athletic overuse injuries and often result from "too much" activity. Both suggest an underlying biomechanical problem, such as poor muscle flexibility or pronation of the feet. I'll also talk about how overuse injuries can be recognized. Parents, coaches, and athletes need to understand overuse injuries because almost every serious athlete will suffer at least one during her sports career.

The mildest form of overuse injury is tendinitis; the most serious is stress fracture. It is important that athletes, their parents, and their coaches understand this continuum. Some overuse injuries at first do not seem serious or painful enough to pull a player from competition, so coaches might say, "Just play through the pain." This is really the wrong advice. With overuse injuries, the more you do, the worse they get. When mild ones are allowed to progress, they can travel along the continuum until they become a full-blown stress fracture.

Tendinitis

Tendinitis means "inflamed tendon," a common overuse injury in growing athletes. Tendons connect muscles to bones. (Ligaments connect bones to each other.) Like most overuse injuries, tendinitis is preventable.

Kevin, a sixteen-year-old basketball player, came in with a three-week history of worsening Achilles pain. He described pain over the

Achilles tendon, the ropelike structure that connects the gastroc-
nemius and soleus (calf) muscles to the calcaneus (heel) bone. Kevin
stated that the pain had intensified over time, and the past two
weeks had been the worst. It increased with activity, particularly
with jumping and landing during basketball practice. He had no rec-
ollection of a specific injury, such as a twisted ankle or having
another player fall on his foot.

Kevin's history is most consistent with tendinitis. Teenagers
are especially susceptible to this injury because their bones are
growing faster than their muscles. Since the growth plate inside
the bone instructs the bone to grow, the muscle is literally stretched
over time, eventually reaching the correct length relative to the
bone. During the teen years, however, and especially during the
growth spurt, the muscle–tendon units are often too short and are
stretched more and more as the bones grow longer. So as kids
grow, they lose flexibility, which is determined by muscle tension, and are much more likely to develop tendinitis. That's
why eight-year-olds can touch their toes much more easily than
fourteen-year-olds can. Given that kids lose flexibility as they grow,
and since we can't and don't want to stop them from growing, the
key to alleviating tendinitis is often to start a good stretching
program.

Keys to Recognizing and Preventing Tendinitis

Early signs of tendinitis are:

- Pain in the tendon.
- Pain that worsens with activity.
- Pain that worsens after sports activity.

To prevent tendinitis:

- Start a muscle-strengthening program before the season starts.
- Stretch and do a good warm-up before every practice and game.
- Recognize the early signs of tendinitis and consult a doctor to pre-
  vent its progression.

I first had Kevin walk down the hall and noticed that he had a slight limp. When I examined his foot and ankle, there was no soreness over the bones; his only site of soreness was over the Achilles tendon. I did not need an X-ray to diagnose Kevin's condition: X-rays show bones, but do not show soft tissue such as tendon, muscle, and cartilage.

Treatment

I told Kevin and his parents that we needed to do two things to help get him better and stay better. First, I pulled him out of basketball for two weeks and sent him to the pool to swim three times a week to keep in shape. Second, I showed him how to use a towel stretch to lengthen his Achilles (see Figure 14). This very helpful stretch should be done by anyone with Achilles pain. The earlier you start this stretch after the pain starts, the quicker the pain will go away. This stretch should be held for 15 seconds, with a minute rest in between. Three repetitions, twice daily, is the best way to stretch. If the Achilles does not improve after a few days, I often send patients to a physical therapist to help with stretching exercises.

Kevin's Achilles tendinitis got better after a two-week rest and good stretching. He returned to the basketball team, kept stretching during the season, and had no further problems.

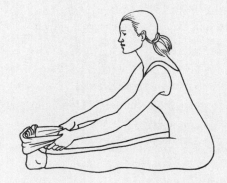

Figure 14.
Achilles stretching.

Stress Fractures

Stress fractures, which are injuries of the bone, are the most serious type of overuse injury. These fractures, which are also known as fatigue fractures, occur when too much stress on the bone creates a site of weakness that eventually causes the cortex (outside) of the bone to begin to crack (see Figure 15). Unlike a regular fracture, a bone break due to a one-time force such as falling on a wrist or crashing into a wall, stress fractures develop over time. They are always serious injuries and require proper diagnosis and treatment to heal, as well as an understanding of why the injury occurred to ensure proper prevention strategies. Stress fractures can happen to any athlete, particularly those whose sport requires them to subject their bones to repeated impact, such as soccer players, runners, figure skaters, and dancers.

Patients with stress fractures often say, "The X-ray I had was normal, so it can't be a stress fracture." They are often surprised when I explain that "stress fracture" is a clinical diagnosis: these fractures frequently don't show up on X-rays, but we can usually tell that it's a stress fracture by the patient's history alone. Sometimes the diagnosis is confirmed with an MRI.

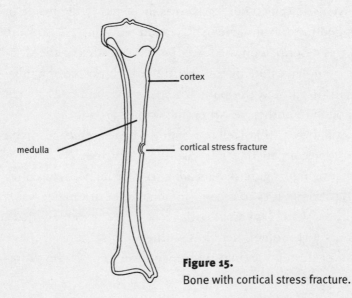

Figure 15.
Bone with cortical stress fracture.

Keys to Recognizing Stress Fractures

- Pain is in one specific part of the body — usually in the feet, legs, or hips — and worsens with activity.
- Point tenderness: pain is in a specific site on the bone.
- Pain worsens over time — first it just hurts a bit with running, then is bad enough so that walking is painful.
- X-rays might be normal, so sometimes an MRI is necessary to diagnose the injury.

Kelly, a thirteen-year-old advanced-level figure skater, is training with her local club. Despite the daily 5:30 a.m. wakeup and the arduous workouts, despite long hours at the rink instead of social events, Kelly never seems to mind the effort — she simply loves to skate, and is anticipating a successful career. Thus far in her skating, she had been injury-free, but she came to me for evaluation of left shin pain that had been bothering her for the past six weeks. Before this pain arose, Kelly had been able to skate for hours; now she had to limit her ice time because the pain in her shin was becoming unbearable. She said, "I'm having a lot of trouble skating, and jumping is especially tough. I don't want to stop skating, but this leg is killing me!" Kelly described her leg pain as localized to the inside of the left shin and most acute when she landed her jumps. A specific area of pain was described on the lower back inside area of the shinbone, a region known as the inferior portion of the posterior medial tibia. She had first noted the pain while skating, but now it had worsened enough to bother her when she walked around.

My first thought was that Kelly probably had a significant injury. Unlike other types of patients, who visit the sports medicine doctor at the slightest twinge, figure skaters are a stoic group who often try to tough it out, sometimes to a fault. In general, performance-sport athletes — figure skaters, gymnasts, dancers — are extremely dedicated to their sport. Sometimes these athletes mistakenly believe they must suffer through an injury for many weeks until the symptoms become severe enough to warrant a visit to a doctor. Usually, this means the pain is so excruciating that they can't perform.

After speaking with Kelly and her parents and getting a better idea of the history of her pain, I examined her leg to find out if there was a focal area of tenderness. She thought she had "shinsplints," a colloquial term used by everyone (doctors, coaches, athletes) to describe shin pain. From her history of focal pain in a bone that worsened with activity, I strongly suspected a stress fracture in Kelly's tibia even before I examined her leg.

First I had Kelly walk down the hall in my office. She was having pain with walking and was limping slightly. When I pushed on the inferior medial portion of the left tibia (the inside part of her shin), she winced. When I asked her to hop on the left leg, again she complained of sharp pain in the back inside part of the lower leg. There were no other focal areas of pain in the lower leg, knee, or hip.

After examining her leg, I examined Kelly's feet to check her biomechanics. When I asked her to stand, I noticed that she "rolled her arches," a condition known as *pronation*. (Figure 16 shows a pronated foot on the right and a normal foot on the left.) Kelly's left foot pronated more than the right. Many people pronate and never have problems, a group known as "happy pronators." But when someone comes in with an overuse injury of a lower extremity (feet, legs, knees, hips) and also pronates, the foot problem needs to be addressed as a factor contributing to the injury.

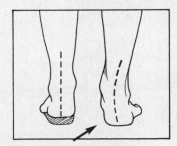

Figure 16.
Pronating (rolling inward) right foot.

Suspecting a stress fracture of the tibia, I sent Kelly for X-rays. The X-rays were normal, as they often are in stress fractures, because the changes in the bone are often not apparent until the bone has either cracked further or fully healed. We want to diagnose the stress fracture earlier to prevent the bone from going on to a full fracture (break).

In this case, because my index of suspicion for stress fracture was very high, despite the normal X-rays, I ordered an MRI (magnetic resonance imaging) of her leg. X-rays simply show a picture of the bone, like a snapshot. MRI uses a powerful magnet to generate a spin-gradient around the affected body part, creating a detailed image. This amazing technology enables us to look inside the body and has significantly changed what we can do. In cases of stress fractures, MRI technology allows us to diagnose them before they show on X-rays. The sooner injuries are detected, the sooner the healing process can begin. In Kelly's case, the stress fracture of the left tibia was clearly demonstrated on the MRI, despite the normal X-rays.

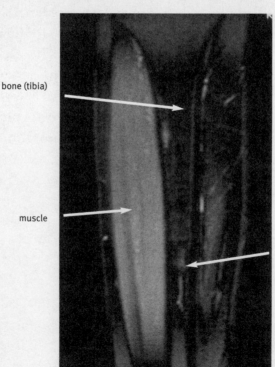

bone (tibia)

muscle

tibial stress fracture

Figure 17.
MRI of tibia.

Treatment

The treatment for stress fracture has multiple steps. The important questions are: (1) Why did this injury occur? (2) What can we
do to make it heal? (3) What can we do to help prevent this injury,
or one like it, from recurring? I emphasize the word *we* here because
effective treatment of any sports injury entails a team of patient, parents, coach, physical therapist, and doctor, all working together to
achieve a positive long-term result.

The answers in Kelly's case:

1. **Why did this injury occur?** Is Kelly training too hard? Are
   the jumps too taxing? Is her body rebelling? The answer here
   seems to be yes to all three. When bones are overstressed by
   pounding or repetitive loading, a stress fracture develops. When
   treating Kelly's injury, the biomechanics of her body, specifically
   the pronation of her left foot, were also addressed. In most cases
   like Kelly's, that is, those involving pronation and an overuse
   injury, the patients should get orthotics (arch supports) for their
   athletic footware. For Kelly, that meant her skates. For soccer
   players or runners, I recommend orthotics for their cleats or
   spikes.

   In general, most patients with simple pronation do well with a
   store-bought, corrective orthotic. These are known as corrective
   because they have a hard fiberglass or plastic bottom that
   corrects the foot's position. If the bottom of the orthotic is
   not hard, the corrective factor is insufficient. Parents should
   bring along the skates, cleats, or spikes to make sure the orthotics
   fit. They should be worn on both feet to avoid a feeling of imbalance. When kids are recovering from a stress fracture, I also have
   them wear orthotics in their street shoes. Sometimes they
   find this so beneficial that they choose to wear them after
   the injury heals. Pronation never disappears, but it is not necessarily always a problem. In general, however, once you have an
   injury-inducing pronation, you are headed toward orthotics for a
   good while. Most of my patients who use orthotics love them

once they start; I know this is the case with my own feet and shins.

Usually, patients with injuries like Kelly's can tolerate the same or increased levels of stress on their legs when their biomechanics are corrected. By correcting her foot problem, Kelly was actually able to skate for longer periods of time than she could tolerate before her injury.

2. **What can we do to make it heal?** Making bones heal takes time, patience, and good biology. Time: Most stress fractures heal within six weeks. Patience: The overaggressive skater who rushes to get back to jumping will delay healing. Good biology: Bones heal with a good diet and normal estrogen levels. (Stress fractures are more common in girls than in boys.)

Diet and hormone levels significantly affect bone healing. Growing teens need 1500 mg of calcium daily. As for hormones, the female estrogen level is highest each month at menstruation. When girls are too skinny, they either never get a period (primary amenorrhea) or lose their period (secondary amenorrhea). In general, females need 15 percent body fat to generate sufficient estrogen to menstruate. If a female doesn't have a period by age fifteen or has gone more than four months without a period after starting menstruation, she should see her doctor. When the estrogen levels are low, bones are prone to developing osteoporosis (low bone density).

Sometimes stress fractures are the only sign that a girl has poor bone density due to low estrogen levels. As I discussed in Chapter 5, the "female athlete triad" is a condition that involves self-starvation (anorexia), absence of menstruation (amenorrhea), and poor bone density (osteoporosis). In a female with a stress fracture, therefore, it is important to ask about both dietary and menstrual history. In Kelly's case, she started her period at age twelve with monthly cycles and she ate a good diet. I therefore attributed the majority of her problems to excessive stress on the bone and poor biomechanics.

3. **What can we do to help prevent this injury, or one like it, from recurring?** We need to examine all the facts to piece together a prevention plan. The amount of jumping, the patient's biomechanics, and her biology are interrelated issues.

Not all children and teenagers are created equal. Different people (kids and adults) have different pain thresholds. Some kids come in to see me when they are just beginning to develop an overuse injury, whereas others come in with a full-blown stress fracture that is cracking through the cortex of the bone. If your child never complains about pain, take any comment about pain seriously. If your child habitually complains about pain a great deal, pay attention to how much the pain is limiting his activity and act accordingly.

Each athlete should also be considered individually in terms of his particular body and the amount of stress he subjects it to. Parents should understand that even if their kid is the only one on the team who's been complaining of shinsplints or knee pain, it's important to have the pain checked out to make sure the tendons and bones are healthy.

Keys to Preventing Stress Fractures

- See a physician when pain develops instead of waiting until the athlete is limping or unable to play.
- If the athlete has had a previous stress fracture, check his biomechanics, activity, and bone density.
- Ensure proper diet (the food pyramid) and calcium intake (more than 1500 mg a day, about three 8-ounce glasses of milk).

As for Kelly, she was "exiled" to the pool for three weeks to work on swimming and deep-water running. I wanted to make sure she kept up her cardiovascular fitness while we waited for her bone to heal. She also bought corrective orthotics at the local sports store and wore them (and continues to wear them) in her shoes and skates. (Wearing them in her shoes helped correct her pronating even when she wasn't skating.) As her pain decreased, she gradually returned to walking, jogging, skating, and finally, seven weeks after being diagnosed, jumping. She has been pain-free for six months and is doing very well.

> ### The Box Score
> - Too much athletics can lead to overuse injury.
> - Overuse injuries are almost always preventable, so the cause needs to be fully investigated.
> - Two very common overuse injuries are tendinitis and stress fracture.
> - See a doctor when pain is in a specific spot and worsens with activity.

Chapter 9

Upper-Body Injuries

ELBOW, BACK, SHOULDER

*Upper-body injuries can occur in many sports. This chapter goes
over some of the common upper-body injuries to help parents
understand them and recognize when to seek further medical attention.*

Elbow Injuries

Elbow injuries are common in sports that involve throwing, and by
far the most common culprit is baseball. When kids throw too
much, or too early, they can injure the growth plate in the elbow,
which, in severe cases, can cause permanent damage.

Little League baseball has been the most proactive organization
in trying to limit the number of "exposure hours," meaning the number of hours a week that an athlete is exposed to a particular sport.
The organization allows kids under the age of twelve to pitch a maximum of six innings a week. There should be no exceptions to this
rule. The case I'm using to illustrate Little League elbow involves a
pitcher who was so good he was on three different teams. He was
throwing only six innings a week for each team, but that added up to
eighteen innings a week. He separated the growth plate in his elbow
and missed an entire year of baseball.

Key Terms

AC separation. Also known as "separated shoulder." It occurs when an athlete falls onto the shoulder, and the ligaments in the acromioclavicular joint are torn.

Axial load injury. Injury resulting from the athlete's landing directly on the shoulder from the side. It is the same mechanism as a clavicle fracture (see below), so with this type of injury the physician must check for clavicle fracture.

Clavicle fracture. Most common fracture in the body. It generally occurs when a player lands directly on the shoulder from the side. This is the same mechanism as an axial load injury (see above).

Discogenic back pain. Back pain due to a bulging disc in the spine. The pain often worsens with bending forward.

Dislocation. When a joint comes fully out of its socket and needs to be put back into place. This is often treated with surgery, especially if there has been more than one episode.

Glenohumeral dislocation. When the shoulder joint comes fully "out of socket" and needs to be put back into place.

Glenohumeral ligament. Ligament that holds the glenohumeral joint together.

Glenohumeral subluxation. Slipping of the main joint in the shoulder (the glenohumeral joint). The joint does not come "out of socket," but slips back into place.

Little League elbow. Pain in the elbow from throwing too much, affecting a young athlete whose growth plates have not yet closed. It can cause permanent damage.

Muscular back pain. Pain along the sides of the spine from muscles that are too weak to function properly. The pain often worsens with torso rotation.

Rotator cuff muscles. Four muscles that work in unison inside the shoulder to provide stability during throwing and overhead sports.

Rotator cuff tendinitis. Inflammation of the rotator cuff tendons. It frequently occurs with swimmers, tennis players, and baseball players.

Shoulder. Joint with greatest range of motion in the body and frequent site of injury for overhead athletes, such as tennis players and baseball players. The shoulder is made up of four joints; the glenohumeral joint and acromioclavicular joint are the most commonly injured in sports.

Spondylolysis. Stress fracture in the spine. The pain often worsens with bending backward.

Subluxation. When a joint slips out of socket, then back into place. This is often treated with rehabilitation to increase muscular strength.

Little League Elbow

Evan, a twelve-year-old baseball pitcher, came with his parents to see me after three months of worsening elbow pain in his right arm. A Little League star, he is competitive, loves to pitch, but has been unable to do so for the past month because the pain keeps getting worse — "It's killing me." He had never been injured before this year.

As I listened to Evan, I grew concerned that his Little League elbow might represent a potentially serious problem: a separation of the growth plate, a condition known as *traction apophysitis*.

Examining Evan's elbow, I noted that he had pain along the inside portion of his elbow, the area known as the *medial epicondyle*. In the medial epicondyle is a growth plate that can be separated from the humerus (upper-arm bone) with repeated throwing. I sent him for an X-ray to evaluate the elbow further. The X-ray showed a separation of the epicondyle from the inside part of the humerus. There are two epicondyles, the medial (inside) and the lateral (outside). In this case, the medial epicondyle was being pulled away, causing elbow pain. (If the force of the muscle actually pulls the bone off, the condition is called a *traction injury*.)

Figure 18.
Flexor muscle in forearm pulling
on medial epicondyle.

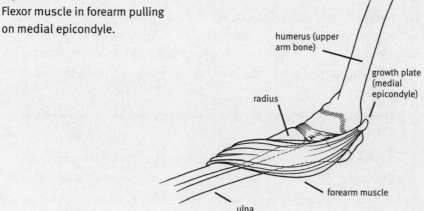

humerus (upper
arm bone)

growth plate
(medial
epicondyle)

radius

forearm muscle

ulna

Little League elbow entails several different types of injuries, all of which cause pain that worsens with too much throwing. Rather than go into detail about specific types of injuries, I think it best for parents and coaches to know when to be concerned about elbow pain.

Elbow pain needs medical attention when:

1. It worsens with throwing.
2. It persists for more than two weeks.
3. The elbow is skeletally immature. (The growth plate there generally doesn't close until about age fourteen).
4. There is swelling in the elbow.
5. The athlete complains of pain for a few weeks.

Evan would not have missed as much baseball if he had consulted a doctor sooner; he had pain for several weeks before he was seen.

Not all cases of Little League elbow are as serious as Evan's. I had him stop throwing for five months, then got him working on exercises in physical therapy to strengthen the muscles on the top and bottom of the forearm. The bone healed, and he was able to return to baseball the next season.

> ## Keys to Preventing Elbow Injuries
> - Do the forearm and shoulder exercises shown in Chapter 7.
> - Comply with the league limits on an individual's throwing.
> - Work on proper throwing mechanics with a pitching or throwing coach.
> - See a physician if pain persists for more than 1 week.

Back Injuries

The back is an interrelated system of muscles, bones, nerves, and discs (which are made of cartilage). Figure 19, an anatomical illustration of the back, shows how all the different parts are interconnected. The key to diagnosing back injuries is knowing that the type of pain an athlete is experiencing indicates which element or structure is involved. Parents need to understand different types of back pain so they can identify the type of problem their children are having and know when to get help.

I will discuss only the most common types of back pain — muscular, discogenic, and bone-related — but there are many other causes of back pain. If back pain persists for more than three weeks, be sure to have a doctor check it out.

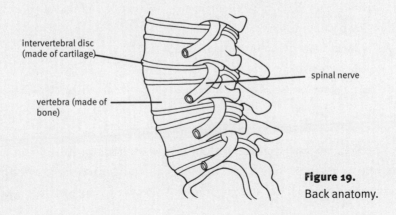

intervertebral disc (made of cartilage)

spinal nerve

vertebra (made of bone)

Figure 19.
Back anatomy.

Muscular Back Pain

Josh, a twelve-year-old hockey player, came in after five weeks of low-back pain. The pain seems most severe when he plays but is also acute after games. Josh said the pain seems to worsen with twisting, especially when he shoots the puck.

Josh's history suggests muscular pain, pain that generally occurs when the back muscles are stressed. This is the most common type of back injury. When I examined him, he had no pain bending forward or backward. His pain worsened with twisting, and he was sore along the sides of his spine.

His X-rays were normal, and I explained to Josh and his parents that I believed he was suffering from muscular back pain, which generally occurs because the muscles in the back are not strong enough to absorb the level of activity across them. In other words, the stronger the muscles, the better able they are to absorb force, such as twisting and lifting. When the muscles are weaker, the same force has a more dramatic effect and can cause muscle tearing, called a *strain*. (Remember: A muscle tear is a *strain*, a ligament tear is a *sprain*.)

Strained muscles tend to go into spasm, and in both kids and adults, a back spasm is what happens when the muscles tighten in the back and become a "knot."

Keys to Recognizing Muscular Back Pain

- There is no radicular (radiating) pain — that is, pain shooting down the back of the leg.
- Pain is along the sides of the spine.
- The pain worsens with twisting.

Treatment

The treatment for muscular back pain depends on the stage of the injury. Back pain is usually due to muscular spasm, so the first step, usually for the first forty-eight hours, is to control the pain.

This can be accomplished with ice, fifteen minutes an hour, and over-the-counter anti-inflammatory medication. Once the initial pain subsides, it's important to start some strengthening exercises to address the injury's underlying cause, such as those designed to strengthen the abdomen and lower back. See pages 168 and 169. An athletic trainer or physical therapist can be very helpful in this regard.

In Josh's case, we iced his back and gave him a few days of anti-inflammatory medicine. He then started to work with his school athletic trainer on some easy strengthening exercises. He was completely better in about three weeks.

Discogenic Back Pain

Alan, a fifteen-year-old football player, came in complaining of two months of back pain, which seemed to worsen with activity, particularly running and lifting weights. He said that when he did any active sports, the pain in his back was so severe it made him wince. Alan also described a shooting pain, down his right leg and into his toes, that sometimes accompanied the back pain.

Listening to him, I was concerned about discogenic back pain, pain resulting from a disc bulging out and pushing on a nerve. This causes pain shooting down the leg and can be really debilitating. With discogenic back pain, the back is so sensitive that the pain can intensify with sneezing or coughing.

Examining Alan's back, I had him stand up and then bend forward. He reported that bending forward caused the shooting pain down his leg.

X-rays were normal, but I sent him for an MRI to see whether he had a herniated (bulging) disc. Herniated discs are usually caused by a tear in the covering of the disc, which can cause part of the disc to leak out and push on the nerve. The shooting pain indicated that a herniated disc was probably pushing on a nerve (see Figure 20), which can sometimes cause permanent nerve damage.

Figure 20.
Herniated disc
pushing on a
spinal nerve.

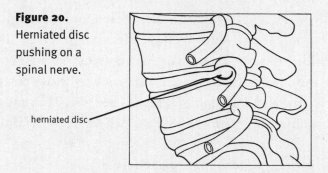

herniated disc

Keys to Recognizing Discogenic Back Pain

- Pain that worsens with bending forward.
- Tingling or shooting pain into the leg or foot.
- Pain that intensifies with coughing or sneezing.

Treatment

Discogenic back pain constitutes about 5 to 10 percent of back pain in teenagers, and about 30 to 40 percent in adults. For teens, we almost always try conservative treatment: using a back brace and physical therapy to help unload pressure off the disc by strengthening the muscles around the spine. This is usually effective. Adults, however, often require steroid injections or sometimes surgery to remove the bulging disc fragment.

In Alan's case, we tried a brace and physical therapy, and he got better in a few weeks. He returned to football one month later and has done well.

Keys to Preventing Discogenic Back Pain

- Develop good muscle strength (do crunches).
- Recognize symptoms early.
- Avoid activities that intensify the symptoms.

Bone-Related Back Pain (Spondylolysis)

Tonia, a fourteen-year-old ballet dancer who loves to dance, is enrolled in a high-level program, and despite her pain, has kept dancing. Her parents brought her to see me because her back pain was worsening; in the past two weeks she had sometimes come home from class crying.

Tonia said there was no tingling or shooting pain into her legs, but that the back pain seemed to worsen when she bent backwards. Figure 21 shows the position Tonia described as causing her the most pain, bending back in a port de bras.

Tonia's description of her back pain immediately made me think about spondylolysis, a stress fracture in the spine common in athletes who load repeated stress on their spine, such as dancers, figure skaters, gymnasts, and volleyball players. The key point in her description of her pain was that it seemed to worsen as she bent backward, a very common condition with spondylolysis-type pain.

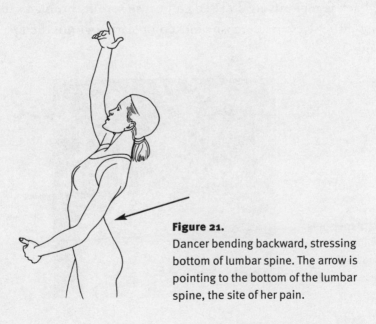

Figure 21.
Dancer bending backward, stressing bottom of lumbar spine. The arrow is pointing to the bottom of the lumbar spine, the site of her pain.

> ## Keys to Recognizing Spondylolysis
> - Back pain that worsens with use.
> - Back pain that worsens with bending backward.
> - Back pain in an athlete in one of the high-risk sports: dance, figure skating, gymnastics, volleyball.

When I examined Tonia, she had no pain bending forward. However, when she bent back she said, "Ow, that's exactly what hurts."

I sent her for X-rays to check for spondylolysis. Her X-rays showed evidence of a stress fracture (shown below in Figure 22). An MRI is sometimes used to make the diagnosis of stress fracure, as with the case of the tibial stress fracure shown in Figure 17, where the X-rays were normal. In Tonia's case, we didn't need an MRI for diagnosis because the X-ray showed the stress fracture.

I explained to Tonia and her parents that the stress fracture in her spine resulted from too much stress on the bone — the bone was actually beginning to crack. Spondylolysis from sports in which the back is repetitively stressed can cause serious problems, especially if the stress fracture isn't picked up early (within the first two months).

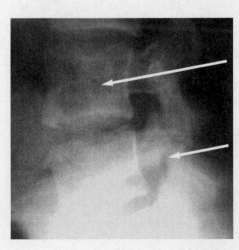

vertebra

spondylolysis
(stress fracture
of spine)

Figure 22.
X-ray of the spine,
showing
spondylolysis
(stress fracture of
the spine).

Tonia was placed in a special brace and kept from dancing. She started physical therapy to strengthen the muscles around her spine. In about six months, the stress fracture healed and she returned to dance. She has done well since.

Shoulder Injuries

Shoulder injuries are common in sports such as tennis, baseball, and swimming that involve overhead motion. Fortunately, most of them, especially overuse injuries, are preventable.

The shoulder has the greatest range of motion of any joint in the body — a full 180 degrees. But this enormous mobility makes it prone to injury because the more movement inside the joint, the more stress on the tissues supporting the joint. Think of a suspension bridge, such as the George Washington Bridge, held together by loose cables. When it shakes in the wind, even more force is needed to hold it in place than when it is stationary. Joints are subject to the same principle. More motion in the joint means more stress on the tissues (particularly muscles) that are trying to hold it in place.

The shoulder is illustrated in Figures 23 and 24. It contains a ball-and-socket-type joint, which is often described as a golf ball sitting precariously on a tee. The humerus (the upper arm bone) is the ball portion of the joint; the scapula (the socket) is the tee. The bones are held together by the glenohumeral ligament, and the small but very important muscles around the joint are called the rotator cuff muscles.

To understand the shoulder, you must understand the concept of shoulder stability. The glenohumeral ligament in the shoulder provides *static stability*, the baseline stability that holds the bones together. The muscles in the shoulder provide *dynamic stability* when the shoulder is in motion. The total stability in the shoulder is equal to the sum of static plus dynamic stability. Some people, by nature,

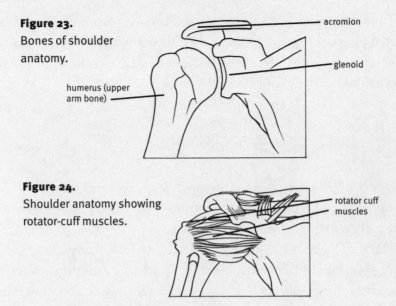

Figure 23.
Bones of shoulder anatomy.

acromion

glenoid

humerus (upper arm bone)

Figure 24.
Shoulder anatomy showing rotator-cuff muscles.

rotator cuff muscles

have very lax ligaments. These are the people who can bend their fingers back and are often double-jointed. Laxity in ligaments any-where means lax ligaments throughout the body. Often, these people have "loose" shoulders that slip out of their sockets. Since they have less static stability, they need to increase their dynamic (muscle) stability to make their shoulder stop slipping. By increasing the dynamic stability, kids and teens can compensate for underlying lack of static stability.

Rotator Cuff Tendinitis

Jenny, a sixteen-year-old swimmer trying to make the state finals, was working hard in practice, extending her yardage to try to increase her speed. She came in to see me with a shoulder that had become increasingly painful over the past few weeks.

Jenny said that at first her shoulder hurt only with swimming, but now it hurt all the time. She said that putting on her shirt in the morning hurt, especially when she raised her arm over her head.

Listening to Jenny, I recognized an overuse injury, an injury that seemed to worsen as she swam more and more. This injury pattern is very common in swimmers and baseball and tennis players.

The keys to her story are a pain that has worsened with time and that seems to worsen with increased stress on the shoulder from swimming. The history is exactly the type we would see in an athlete who is putting too much stress on rotator cuff muscles that are not strong enough to stand up to the repetitive force of swimming.

When I examined Jenny's shoulder, I saw that she had pain when lifting her arm over her head, a type of motion called *abduction*. When she tried to raise her arm to the side, she described a "pinching" pain in the shoulder.

X-rays of Jenny's shoulder were normal, and I explained to her parents that I believed she had developed an overuse injury in her shoulder called rotator cuff tendinitis.

As discussed in Chapter 8, irritation of a tendon is known as tendinitis; we see it frequently in several areas of the body, including the Achilles tendon and the rotator cuff. The rotator cuff muscles provide dynamic stability to the shoulder; they are responsible for keeping the golf ball (the head of the humerus) centered on the tee (the scapula). When an athlete asks too much of the rotator cuff, putting demands on the muscles that are greater than the force they are able to produce, the tendon (the connection between muscle and bone) can become irritated. Instead of the muscle dissipating the force of joint motion, the tendon is forced to do the work. Over time, the tendon, which is less well designed to absorb force than muscle is, will become inflamed.

Treatment

The keys to treating rotator cuff tendinitis are (1) relative rest from sport and (2) aggressive strengthening. Relative rest means that if swimming is causing the pain, the athlete should not swim for about a week. I say "relative rest" because it's very important for the athlete to stay fit. Cardiovascular fitness declines quickly with inactivity. We estimate that every day that an athlete doesn't exercise, she loses 2 to 3 percent of overall fitness. Exercise biking and running are often helpful substitutes for swimming because they keep the body in shape and don't use the shoulder much. A combination of anti-inflammatory medicine and rest is often helpful to get an athlete to a pain-free state. This means that the shoulder should not hurt when it is moved or raised overhead. After the shoulder quiets down with medicine and rest, the next and most important step is strengthening exercises.

When undertaking a rotator cuff strengthening program after injury, it's important to work with a physical therapist. Shoulder rehabilitation is tricky; if not done properly, you can make things worse instead of better. Start a strengthening program quickly, usually within a few days of the onset of pain, because muscles atrophy (lose strength) when they are not used. By taking time off from using the shoulder, an athlete will actually lose strength, and although the pain will subside during the time off, it will quickly reappear when the athlete starts swimming or serving tennis balls again because the weakness in the muscles underlying the pain will have increased.

In Jenny's case, I kept her out of the pool, put her on a five-day course of anti-inflammatory medicine, and started her in physical therapy right away. Within two weeks she was feeling much better and was swimming again three weeks after her injury.

Keys to Recognizing Rotator Cuff Tendinitis

- Pain that worsens with activity.
- Pain when lifting shoulder overhead.
- Pain with overhead sports (swimming, baseball, tennis, other racquet sports).

It's much preferable to prevent rotator cuff problems than to treat them after they have occurred. The best way to prevent rotator cuff tendinitis is through an aggressive strengthening program. The basics of such a program are illustrated below. Athletes with a history of shoulder problems such as Jenny's should start on a strengthening program of three times a week, six weeks before the season starts. During the season, they should be strengthening at least once a week in addition to normal workouts. Ideally, the swimming,

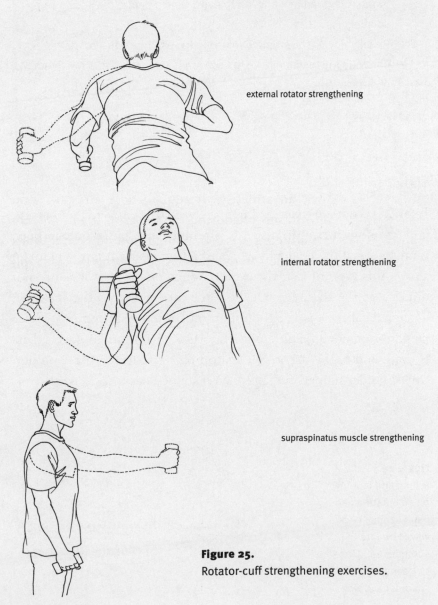

external rotator strengthening

internal rotator strengthening

supraspinatus muscle strengthening

Figure 25.
Rotator-cuff strengthening exercises.

tennis, or baseball coach will add strengthening to the practice time to make sure all the athletes actively participate.

> ## Keys to Preventing Rotator Cuff Tendinitis
> - Start strengthening early, six to eight weeks before the sports season begins.
> - Be diligent; do the strengthening exercises three times a week.
> - Continue the regimen once the season is under way, at a minimum of once a week.

Shoulder Instability

Jason, a seventeen-year-old rugby player, came to see me one day complaining of pain in his right shoulder. Evidently he had been running down the field and fell, landing on his right arm. Figure 26 shows this type of fall: the athlete lands on an arm or hand, not directly on the shoulder, but the force carries up into the shoulder. The medical term is "a fall onto an outstretched extremity." These falls are common in high-contact sports such as football, soccer, basketball, and rugby. Jason felt a slipping sensation in his shoulder: "My shoulder slipped out, and then it slipped back in," he said.

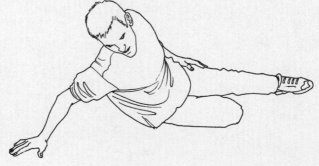

Figure 26.
Falling and landing on an outstretched hand sends shock waves up into the shoulder and leads to a sensation of the shoulder slipping.

Jason was describing shoulder instability, the term used when the shoulder (glenohumeral joint) slips. There are two grades of instability: *subluxation*, a slip when the shoulder doesn't fully come out of socket, and a *dislocation*, when the shoulder joint comes all the way out and needs to be put back into the socket. Jason described subluxation.

As I explained earlier, the total stability of the shoulder results from the combined stability of both the ligaments and the muscles. When the ligaments are loose, the shoulder is prone to slipping, either subluxation or dislocation. When a patient suffers a subluxation episode, he needs to understand that it is due to the lack of ligamentous stability and he is prone to repeat episodes. Subluxation can go on to become dislocation, because over time and repeated subluxation episodes, the ligaments stretch. The shoulder actually becomes looser and more prone to dislocation.

Examining Jason's shoulder convinced me that he had suffered a glenohumeral subluxation episode. He had pain when moving the shoulder overhead and pain along the front part of his shoulder. I examined his shoulder for ligamentous instability and found that his shoulder was slipping.

Treatment

Advising him that without treatment he would probably experience repeat episodes and risk dislocation, I sent Jason to a physical therapist to begin an aggressive muscle-strengthening program designed to make his rotator cuff muscles move more effectively (see Figure 25, page 203). Within four weeks, he was doing much better. He returned to sports six weeks after injury and has done well since.

Keys to Recognizing Shoulder Instability
- Slipping sensation in shoulder.
- Pain is sometimes associated with tingling in hands and fingers.
- Athlete often has a previous history of slipping episodes.

Separated Shoulder

Paul, a sixteen-year-old soccer player, came in with a shoulder injury. When he fell during a game, landing directly on his right shoulder, he immediately felt pain over the top of his shoulder. His shoulder had never been injured before.

The mechanism of Paul's injury (the way he sustained it) is pictured in Figure 27. When an athlete lands directly on the outside of the shoulder, the injury is known as an *axial load injury* to the shoulder.

Unlike Jason, who talked about a "slipping sensation" in the shoulder from landing on an outstretched arm, Paul described an acute pain on the top of his shoulder resulting from falling on the side of his shoulder joint.

An axial load injury is the most common way to injure the clavicle (collarbone — the most commonly fractured bone in the body) and, in particular, the acromioclavicular joint (AC joint) on the top part of the shoulder.

Paul's examination confirmed pain just over the AC joint. There was no tenderness over the clavicle, which would have raised suspicion for a clavicle fracture. X-rays of the shoulder were normal. I diagnosed Paul with a grade I AC separation (shoulder separation). Shoulder separation is very common, especially in high-contact sports like football, rugby, and soccer. The injury occurs

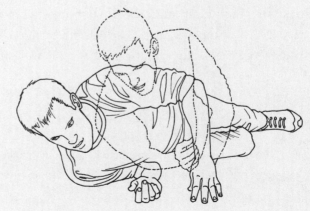

Figure 27.
Falling directly on the shoulder can cause the shoulder to separate.

along a spectrum: the most common and mildest, called grade I, gives a normal X-ray; the least common and most serious, grade V, involves a fracture and requires surgery.

I put the arm in a sling for comfort for a few days. Paul began using his shoulder for activities in a week, and was back to full activity four weeks after injury.

Keys to Recognizing and Treating AC Joint Injuries

- Mechanism of injury is axial loading.
- Take X-rays to make sure the clavicle isn't fractured.
- Have injury evaluated by doctor to establish grade.
- Use a sling for comfort in grade I and II injuries.
- Return to sports is generally about 1 month in grade I and II injuries.

Remember: A book can only give guidelines. Nothing can substitute for an individual examination, so it's important to see your doctor to confirm what you've learned from my discussion here.

The Box Score

- Persistent pain (longer than two weeks) in the upper body is usually a signal of muscle weakness.
- Ignoring muscle weakness can lead to more serious injuries.
- Ligamentous laxity (looseness) can predispose overhead sport athletes to develop shoulder injuries.
- Strengthening the relevant muscles either on your own before injury or with a physical therapist once the injury has occurred is key to preventing future injuries.

Chapter 10

Lower-Body Injuries

ANKLES AND KNEES

Except for arm wrestling, I can't think of a sport that doesn't
depend on the legs, and lower-body injuries — ankles and knees —
are the most common types of sports injuries that I see in my office.
This chapter will explain these injuries and teach parents how to
recognize injury patterns. I cover ACL (anterior cruciate ligament)
injuries in some detail because we are seeing more of these than
ever before. I also discuss strategies to help prevent ankle and
knee injuries and reduce the risk of recurrence.

The Slightly Unstable Ankle

The ankle is the most commonly injured joint in the body. At one time or another during the sports career of their young athletes, most families have had to deal with ankle injuries. So recognizing how they occur and knowing what to do when they occur is very important for parents.

The ankle is a very complicated joint that moves in four directions: up, down, and side to side. As a result it is inherently unstable, and, not surprisingly, ankle injuries are a common occurrence in

208

Key Terms

Anterior cruciate ligament (ACL). The main ligament in the knee, the ACL runs inside the intercondylar notch in the knee and holds the femur and tibia together when the knee twists. The ACL is the ligament that most commonly needs surgery for repair.

ACL rupture. Complete tearing of the ACL. The ligament snaps like a rubber band. This injury is at least three to four times more common in females than in males.

Ankle. The most commonly injured joint in the body.

Anterior talofibular ligament (ATFL). The most commonly sprained ligament in the body. It is located on the outside (lateral) part of the ankle.

Articular cartilage. The cartilage covering the bones in the joints, such as the knee. When the articular cartilage surface wears down, doctors call it osteoarthritis, which is usually what people refer to when they say they have arthritis.

Deltoid ligament. The thickest ligament in the ankle, it is located on the inside (medial) of the ankle. To injure this ligament requires significant force.

Eversion. Rolling outward on the ankle. It is less common than inversion but more serious.

Intercondylar notch. The space where the cruciate ligaments (ACL/PCL) are located.

Inversion. The classic type of "rolling over," or rolling inward on the ankle.

Ligament. Connective tissue that ties bones together.

Medial collateral ligament/lateral collateral ligament (MCL/LCL). Responsible for stabilizing the sides of the knee, the collateral ligaments provide stability for side-to-side movements.

Meniscus. The cartilage plates in the knee between the femur (thigh bone) and tibia (lower leg bone).

MRI (magnetic resonance imaging). A computer-generated image that uses a magnetic field to show the soft tissues (tendon, ligament, muscle, and cartilage) and their injuries.

Patella. The medical term for kneecap.

Patellofemoral knee pain. The most common type of knee pain. It occurs in the front of the knee, underneath the patella.

RICE (Rest, Ice, Compression, Elevation). Treatment of injured ankle or knee during first 24 to 48 hours after injury.

Sprain. Partial tearing of a ligament.

Strain. Muscle injury; partial tearing of the muscle.

X-Ray. An X-ray shows bones but not soft tissue such as tendon, ligament, muscle, and cartilage.

most sports. Every weight-bearing movement we make, whether walking, running, jumping, or kicking, exerts tremendous force across the ankles and knees. Sports increase the amount of force, not only through the repetition of the activity but also through the power behind the movement.

The ankle consists of the bones of the lower leg, the tibia and fibula, as well as the talus and calcaneus bones in the foot. Figure 28, on page 211, shows the ankle and how the ligaments connect the bones together. There are three main ligaments on the outside part of the ankle, and these are the most commonly injured ligaments in the body.

Inversion Injury: "Rolling Over on the Ankle"

Jamie, a fourteen-year-old soccer player, came in two days after running down the field, stepping in a hole, and "rolling over" on his ankle, with the sole of the foot facing inward. His parents took him home, applied ice, and waited to see what would happen. The ankle swelled that night, and they brought him in two days later.

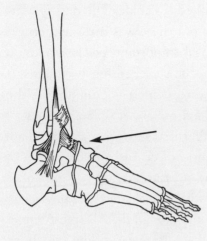

Figure 28.
Outside view of the ankle. The arrow is pointing to an ATFL ligament tear.

The mechanism of the injury that Jamie described is an *inversion*, the most common type of ankle injury. The tibia, the inside bone in the ankle, is about 1 centimeter shorter than the fibula, the outside ankle bone, so that it's much easier to roll over on the ankle from the outside in (inversion) than from the inside out (eversion). The inversion mechanism is pictured in Figure 29.

When I examined Jamie's ankle, I paid particular attention to how he was walking. He was limping a bit as he walked down the hall, and I explained to his parents that limping in a child or teen should always be investigated, especially if it persists beyond one or two days. Two days after his injury, Jamie was limping only slightly.

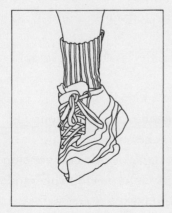

Figure 29.
Inversion injury to the ankle.

After watching him walk, I examined his ankle. The outside (lateral) part of his ankle was swollen, but there was little tenderness when I pushed on the fibula. This was important, because pain on the bone is always something physicians take seriously. In kids, it can represent a growth-plate fracture, which is common in the ankle. Parents are not expected to diagnose growth-plate injuries, of course, but it's important to remember that kids with growth-plate fractures will often continue to limp noticeably and complain of ongoing pain for several days. If pain persists beyond two days after an ankle sprain, be sure to have the athlete evaluated by a physician.

Continuing to examine Jamie's ankle, I found that the most tender area was at the point just in front of the outside part of the anklebone (lateral malleolus), over the most commonly sprained ligament in the body, the anterior talofibular ligament (ATFL). Accordingly, I diagnosed Jamie with a sprained ligament, in this case a sprained ATFL.

Treatment

As previously noted, ankle sprains are very common, and more than 80 percent of them involve the ATFL. But the most common reason that athletes consult a physician for sprained ankles is that they have sprained the ankle before and have not completely rehabilitated from the initial injury. The key to treating Jamie was not just to treat the present injury, but to develop a strengthening program so that this injury does not recur.

The first step to treating ankle injury is applying RICE in the first twenty-four to forty-eight hours. RICE means

- Rest. That is, stay off the ankle. Rest is the most important component of RICE.
- Ice. This will diminish swelling and help control the pain. Apply ice to the injured area for fifteen minutes every hour. Use a regular ice pack or a bag of frozen vegetables.
- Compression. An Ace wrap to apply gentle compression on the ankle will help reduce swelling. Don't wrap the bandage too tightly — just enough to supply a gentle squeeze.

• Elevation. This prevents the swelling from "pooling" in the ankle when walking. Keeping the ankle elevated (on a couch, chair, or pillow) can reduce swelling in the first twenty-four hours.

RICE doesn't mean the athlete should sit on the couch and not move for two days, but just that when sitting, it's best to keep the ankle elevated instead of down.

After the first forty-eight hours, Jamie's ankle felt better. In most mild to moderate ankle sprains, the sooner you start physical therapy, the sooner you're able to return to activity. In Jamie's case, I sent him directly to physical therapy from my office. The physical therapists started him on a strengthening program, initially to decrease swelling and pain in the ankle through *isometric* exercises (pushing the ankle against a hard surface), and then the next week, to build strength through *isotonic* exercises (strengthening with the joint moving).

After one week, Jamie was well enough to start playing again with his ankle taped. By three weeks, he had recovered completely. Once the ankle feels better, the absolute essential is to prevent the injury from recurring by starting a strengthening program (see Figure 31, page 216). Even if you don't seek treatment from a doctor for an ankle sprain (many people don't), be sure to start a preventive ankle-strengthening program. This can be done shortly after the injury, or even many months later.

Eversion Injury: Rolling the Ankle "the Other Way"

Seth, a seventeen-year-old football player, saw me four days after suffering a bad ankle sprain. Running down the field and trying to avoid a tackle, he had cut to his right and rolled on his ankle "the other way, from the inside out." This is a good description of what is otherwise known as an *eversion injury*.

Seth said this eversion injury hurt "a lot" and that it was the first time he had sprained his ankle this way (his previous sprains were inversion injuries). The mechanism of Seth's injury is pictured in Figure 30, which follows.

Figure 30.

Eversion injury to the ankle.

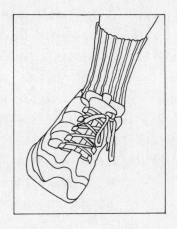

Seth was limping noticeably as he walked down the hall. When I examined his ankle and leg, the majority of swelling and pain was on the inside part of the ankle, just beneath the medial malleolus (inside anklebone). I took extra care to examine his lower leg as well as his ankle, since eversion injuries are associated with fractures of the fibula, the thin bone on the outside part of the lower leg. Fortunately, Seth had no tenderness in the lower leg; most of his pain was on the inside part of the ankle. X-rays of the ankle were normal. I diagnosed a sprain of the deltoid ligament, the ligament on the inside (medial) part of the ankle.

Deltoid ligament injuries are common with eversion injuries. What parents, coaches, and kids need to know is that eversion injury is much more serious than inversion injury and should be evaluated by a doctor. The deltoid ligament is much stronger than the ligaments on the outside part of the ankle; it is three layers thick while the ATFL is only one layer thick. Thus deltoid ligament sprains are much more serious because it takes more force to injure the inside part of the ankle than the outside.

Treatment

The treatment for deltoid ligament injuries in the first forty-eight hours is RICE, the same as for inversion injuries. However, unlike ATFL injuries, which can sometimes be effectively treated at home, deltoid injuries should always be seen by a doctor. Furthermore, since these injuries are more serious, they take much longer to heal, usually two to three months before an athlete is pain-free.

It is almost always the rule to start an athlete with a history of a deltoid sprain in physical therapy, as this injury takes longer to heal and requires more hands-on work. I started Seth in a physical therapy program and he worked hard, never skipping a day and concentrating on the exercises when he was doing them. He was back on the football field six weeks after injury.

Prevention

The most important thing I tell patients with sprained ankles is "If you have done this once, you are much more likely to do it again. Let's focus on preventive strengthening for the next six weeks so this doesn't become a habit."

Usually, the athlete can start a strengthening program about forty-eight hours after the injury has occurred. If the ankle is still painful, it's best to see a doctor first, and also to start a formal physical therapy program instead of working on your own. But in the case of a mild sprain, in which the ankle is much less sore after the first couple of days, strengthening on your own is appropriate. These exercises are also tremendously helpful for kids who have had a history of rolling their ankle year after year. By starting the program I outline below before the season begins, the likelihood of repeat ankle injury is greatly reduced.

This program takes six weeks to make a difference in function, so starting six weeks before the season is key. Muscle stability takes time to develop; it doesn't just happen overnight.

Take an Ace bandage, tie the ends together to make a loop, then hook one end around a table leg or have someone hold it. If you want to get really fancy, go to a local surgical supply store and buy a three-foot-long piece of Thera-Band, the type of resistance band used in physical therapy. The other end goes around the ball of the foot. The ankle is slowly inverted (rolled inward) against resistance with the Ace bandage on the inside of the foot, and then everted

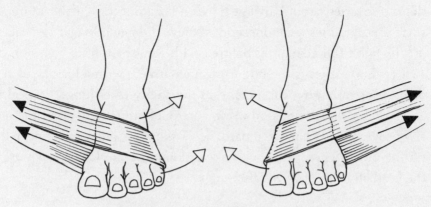

Figure 31. Ankle-strengthening program.

(rolled outward) with the Ace bandage on the outside of the foot. I recommend three sets of 15 repetitions on each foot in each direction, done slowly and deliberately against resistance. It's important not to rush through these exercises, but to take enough time to make a difference. Each repetition should take about five seconds. Move slowly and deliberately against the resistance to strengthen the muscle. By doing three sets of 15 repetitions of resisted inversion and eversion, an ankle that has been repeatedly injured during the sports season will function much better, and the chance of reinjury is greatly reduced.

Keys to Ankle Injuries

- Recognize the mechanism (inversion vs. eversion).
- Remember that eversion injuries are usually more serious.
- Be wary of growth-plate injuries in kids under age 14, especially if the pain persists on the outside part of the ankle for more than 48 hours.
- Use RICE for first 1 to 2 days.
- See a physician if the pain persists for more than 48 hours or if the ankle looks bad (swollen, blue, bruised).
- Once the pain has lessened, develop a preventive strengthening program to keep the injury from recurring.

The Amazing Knee

The knee is amazing. The most powerful joint in the body, and the one that bears more weight than any other, the knee routinely sustains forces of six to seven times body weight. Constructed with extraordinary efficiency, the knee is capable of bending to 160 degrees, twisting 30 degrees in both directions, and withstanding tremendous impact. Knees allow us to run, change direction rapidly, and jump high in the air. Although very strong and stable, knees are frequently injured. When knee injuries happen to kids, teens, or adults, the thought is often the same: "Is this injury going to need surgery and ruin my sports career?" Fortunately, most knee injuries don't require surgery and heal within a few weeks.

Knee Anatomy

Bones

The innermost layer of the knee is made up of bones. The knee bones include the femur, the strongest bone in the body (also known as the thighbone), the lower leg bone known as the tibia, and the kneecap, or patella. Since the knee bears more weight than any other joint in the body, the bones around the knee are hard and durable. Generally speaking, only a very forceful injury such as a high-speed collision will fracture a bone in the knee, and such injuries are rare in sports such as basketball, baseball, or soccer. Sports-related knee fractures usually result from the bones around the knee being struck hard by football helmets or similar objects. For example, I have seen a snowboarder who fractured his patella by ramming his knee into a tree at high speed and a hockey player who fractured his tibia by crashing into the bench. Even in contact sports such as football and hockey, however, any fracture of the bones in the knee is an extremely rare occurrence.

Ligaments

The bones inside the knee move in unison due to the four ligaments that connect them. When the femur twists, the tibia twists; when the femur straightens, the tibia straightens. Much like four cables connecting two pieces of wood, the four knee ligaments connect the tibia and femur and keep them working together.

The four ligaments in the knee are named for their position:

Anterior cruciate ligament (ACL) — runs inside the knee, back to front.

Posterior cruciate ligament (PCL) — runs inside the knee, front to back.

Medial collateral ligament (MCL) — runs along the inside of the knee.

Lateral collateral ligament (LCL) — runs along the outside of the knee.

A partial tear of a ligament is called a *sprain* and a complete tear is called a *rupture*. Since the force required to sprain or rupture a ligament is much less than the force required to fracture a bone, ligament injuries occur much more commonly than bone injuries. Unlike fractures, which almost always occur from a traumatic force,

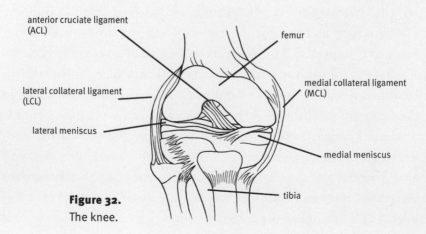

Figure 32.
The knee.

ligament injuries can occur with or without contact. Examples of contact ligament injuries I have seen include a rugby player who was struck from the outside of her knee by another player's head and a baseball player struck on the inside of his knee by a sliding baserunner. Both of these athletes sustained ligament sprains. More commonly, however, knee ligament injuries are noncontact, resulting from a twisting-type force.

The young athlete who twists a knee can injure the ligaments without damaging the bone. In looking at ligament injuries, the most helpful diagnostic tool is the MRI (magnetic resonance imaging). Unlike X-ray, which shows only bone, MRI uses a high-intensity magnetic field, which easily shows not only the difference between bone, soft tissue (such as cartilage, ligament, and tendon), and joint fluid, but also injury to these parts.

Cartilage (meniscus)

Between the tibia and femur are two types of cartilage that serve as shock absorbers in the knee: the meniscus (the cartilage between the bones) and the articular cartilage (which covers the bones). Cartilage provides both cushion and structural support to the knee. Like ligaments, cartilage is visible only on an MRI. Young athletes can injure cartilage in the knee through twisting. As with ligament injuries, the sports that require twisting in the knee such as skiing and soccer carry the highest incidence of cartilage injuries.

Meniscus Cartilage Repair. Repair of the meniscus cartilage is done by sewing the torn ends together. This is usually done on an outpatient basis. Adolescents, because they heal better than adults (age slows healing), are much more likely to be candidates for meniscus repair; adults often have the torn piece of meniscus taken out. It is generally preferable to repair torn meniscus if possible because once the meniscus is taken out, a patient is more likely to develop osteoarthritis as an adult. In general, young athletes are on crutches for five weeks and are back to full sports participation by about four months.

How can I tell if a knee injury is serious?

Listen to your child. If the injury sounds bad, looks bad, or is causing him or her to limp, get further help. Here are some other important indicators:

- **Swelling** — Swelling in the knee, especially within an hour of injury, suggests the injury may be serious.
- **Activity** — Generally, children stop playing when something really wrong has happened. Continuing to run around is usually a good sign.
- **Instability** — A serious knee injury will often cause the sensation of instability or looseness in the knee. If a young athlete reports instability, consult a doctor.
- **Popping sensation** — If the injured athlete reports hearing or feeling a *pop* in his knee at the moment of injury, there's a strong chance of serious injury. Consult a doctor.

Where should I go to have my child's knee evaluated?

Many high schools have athletic trainers who offer the first line of treatment for sports injuries. For acute injuries, emergency rooms can use X-rays to tell if there is a fracture in the knee. Afterward, a sports medicine physician, someone trained to evaluate sports injuries, is often consulted.

Do knee injuries in children cause arthritis when they're older?

Generally, no. Only the rare injury, such as a very bad cartilage injury, causes arthritis in knees during adult life. In fact, exercise is a great way to help all bones grow stronger.

What sports have the highest incidence of knee injuries?

Those that involve twisting place the knee at greatest risk: soccer, basketball, football, lacrosse, rugby, volleyball, and skiing.

As is the case with ankle injuries, knee injuries are best understood by evaluating the mechanism of injury. Falling on a knee and hurting the kneecap results in a different type of injury than twisting the knee. Though both will produce complaints of pain in the knee, their prognoses are very different. The mechanism of injury — the events that cause the injury — is the most effective indicator in determining the severity of an injury.

Twisting Injuries

A general rule for parents: *Twisting injuries are potentially serious.*

Twisting injuries, the most serious type of knee injuries, most often do not involve contact with another player. For this reason, they can appear falsely innocuous. In this type of injury, the foot is fixed to the floor and the athlete twists the body above a planted foot. Figure 33 shows the most common scenario for ACL injury, the twisting injury where the foot is planted. Twisting can also cause the meniscus cartilage to tear. Both types of injury usually require surgery.

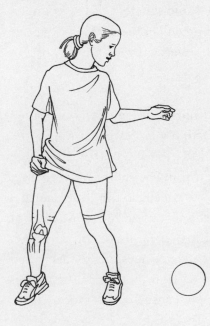

Figure 33.
Soccer player suffering twisting injury to right knee with planted foot.

Footwear

With advances in footwear for sports such as basketball and soccer, and in ski technology, including better bindings and parabolic skis, the twisting type of knee injury has become much more common over the past ten years. The reason is simple. As footwear holds the foot and ankle more firmly in place, the knee is subject to torsion forces that were previously encountered by the ankle. Years ago, ankle sprains were more common as ankles tended to give way with torsion forces. Now with the ankle and foot more firmly secured due to improved technology, the knee is often injured instead. Studies investigating the optimal type of footwear for sports such as basketball are currently under way; they aim to develop shoes that protect the ankle while decreasing the friction between the sole and the floor. This style should be available within the next few years.

With skis, it's important that the bindings be set for the weight and ability of the child who will use them. I've seen several children with ACL tears from bindings that didn't release. This often occurs when a heavier, older sibling passes down skis; the bindings are most likely set for the weight and ability of the child who used them last, even though both children may have the same size feet. If the younger, lighter sibling twists a knee, the binding will not release. This type of twisting injury is potentially serious but very preventable.

Age

ACL tears and other twisting injuries are more common in teenagers than in younger kids. As thigh muscles get stronger, the force they generate increases as kids grow, so that the force absorbed by the knee with a twisting injury increases with age. Before puberty, twisting injuries in the knee result in little damage. When a little kid twists her knee, the force exerted is usually not strong enough to tear any of the soft tissues (ligament, cartilage, tendon, muscle). As puberty begins and continues, the force exerted increases, so that the same twisting motion that is of little consequence to the eight-year-old child can cause a much more serious injury in the thirteen-year-old.

Gender

Studies of both college and high school athletes indicate that ACL tear is at least three to four times more common in females, especially those involved in soccer and basketball. The reasons for this are not yet fully understood, though the two most popular theories suggest that the intercondylar notch is narrower in females, giving the ligament less room to maneuver with a twisting motion. When a sudden twist occurs, the ligament is torn. Figure 34 shows the intercondylar notch, the tunnel through which the cruciate ligaments run.

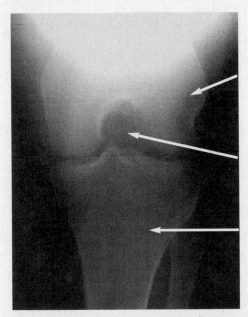

femur

intercondylar notch

tibia

Figure 34.
X-ray of the knee showing intercondylar notch.

Another possible reason that ACL injuries are more common in females is a difference in muscle distribution. Athletic females tend to build up quadriceps muscles (the front muscles of the thigh) more than hamstring muscles (the muscles behind the thigh). In contrast, athletic males tend to build even amounts of both quadriceps and hamstring muscles. When faced with a sudden twist, the female athlete tends to create an anterior force — that is, her twisting motion or sudden stopping motion can cause the upper leg to shift forward because the quads are pulling against a weaker hamstring force. Thus prevention of ACL injuries in girls might be linked to the better distribution of force between the quads and the hamstrings.

Potential Injuries from a Twisting Mechanism

- ACL tear
- Meniscus cartilage tear

Prognosis: Poor short-term; both will probably require surgery. Favorable long-term; athletes usually return to full competition 6 to 8 months after surgery.

Tearing the ACL: A Case Study

Andrew, age eighteen, the captain of the basketball team, came in to see me on crutches two days after suffering a knee injury.

"I was playing in the game and had just pulled down a rebound. No one was around me and I turned to throw the ball upcourt. I felt a *pop* in my left knee and a sharp, sudden pain, like my knee exploded inside. I felt the pain inside, deep inside my knee. I didn't have to look down to know it was something bad!

"I tried to run up the court but the knee kept shifting underneath me. Even though I was able to run, the bones inside my knee felt like they were moving around; the knee felt loose. I knew something was really, really wrong, worse than any of the other injuries I'd had before. I came out of the game and iced my knee. It swelled a bit but didn't hurt too much when I kept it still. After ten minutes or so, the pain went away.

"My parents took me to the hospital emergency room, where they took an X-ray of my knee. They told me that the X-ray was normal, gave me crutches, and told me to see a sports medicine doctor in a couple of days."

Three key points in Andrew's story told me this knee injury was serious: the swelling of the knee, his inability to continue playing after the injury occurred, and the mechanism of injury. The planting, twisting, noncontact injury is the hallmark of an ACL tear. Andrew's description of a "pop" and the associated sensation of a deep pain inside the knee made me even more suspicious of an ACL tear.

I tested Andrew's ACL using a maneuver called the Lachman test: the examiner puts stress on the tibia and femur to see whether the bones have excessive movement. In Andrew's case, unfortunately, they did.

Since I knew the X-rays were normal, I didn't bother repeating them. X-rays don't show ligament or cartilage injuries. An MRI obtained that evening showed a torn ACL (Figures 35 and 36). There was no associated articular or meniscus cartilage damage.

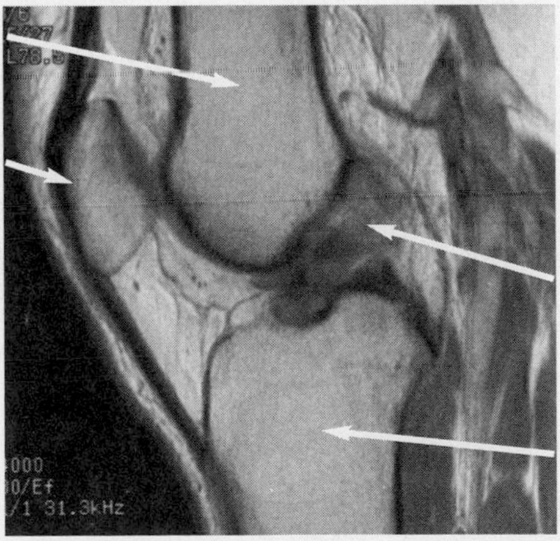

femur

patella
(kneecap)

Figure 35.
MRI of the knee
showing a torn ACL.

torn ACL

tibia

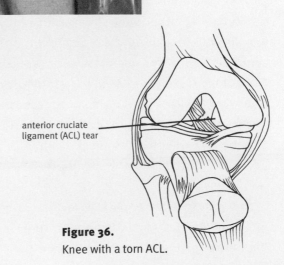

anterior cruciate
ligament (ACL) tear

Figure 36.
Knee with a torn ACL.

(Articular cartilage covers the surface of joints; meniscus cartilage is the cartilage between the femur and the tibia.)

Treatment

I broke the news to Andrew and his parents the next day. It's extremely difficult telling a high school senior that he has played his last high school game. Most families take it very hard. On the one hand, they know "It's not cancer, it's just a sports injury. I should be happy this is all I'm hearing." On the other hand, athletics is an integral part of many kids' lives. When this is taken away for a while, it's very tough. I always tell parents to watch out for depression after major injuries. In such cases, it's important to keep kids as active as they can be, both physically and mentally. This is best accomplished through a carefully designed physical therapy program, supervised by a trained professional to ensure the correct quality and intensity of activity.

Andrew served as an assistant coach for the rest of the season. One month after his ACL tear, he had his knee repaired through a process called ACL reconstructive surgery. He now has a new ligament and is strengthening his knee in physical therapy, rehabilitating the muscles around the knee and preparing for his college basketball career.

ACL Reconstruction. ACL reconstruction is usually done on an outpatient basis (meaning the patient goes home the same day). Anesthesia can be either general (meaning fully sleeping) or through a spinal block (meaning the legs are temporarily put to sleep). The actual repair involves a graft of tissue, usually from the person's own body. This is known as an autograft. Most often, this tissue is taken from the patellar tendon. (In some cases the surgeon will use tissue from a cadaver; this is called an allograft.) Patients are usually on crutches for three to four weeks following surgery and are back to full sports participation by six months.

Prevention of Twisting Knee Injuries

Young athletes can do two things to lessen the likelihood of twisting injuries: weight-train and choose the proper shoes. Since ACL tear might be related to the disproportionate strength of the ham-strings and quadriceps muscles, females involved in twisting sports should work on hamstring strengthening. I believe that this is the single most important preventive step female athletes can take to reduce their risk of ACL injury. This type of strengthening is best accomplished through hamstring curls while lying on the stomach or elbows (see Figure 37).

Do three sets of 15 repetitions on each leg, using 10-pound ankle weights. When this amount of weight is no longer difficult to repeat for three sets, increase the weight by 5-pound increments. These exercises should be started six weeks before the sports season begins.

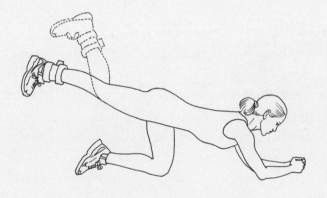

Figure 37. Hamstring-curl exercise to prevent ACL injury.

Lateral Contact Injury

Another common mechanism of knee injury is the lateral contact injury, caused by a force striking the knee from the outside. These injuries commonly occur in contact sports such as football, lacrosse, rugby, and soccer.

Zack, age fifteen, came to my office after suffering an injury during a soccer game that morning. He was running down the field with the ball when another player hit his knee from the out-side. Though the injury occurred from the outside, Zack felt pain in the inside of his knee. The knee did not swell. The history and exam led me to diagnose a sprain of the medial collateral ligament (MCL).

Figure 38.
A lateral-contact knee injury occurs when a player
is struck on the outside of the knee.

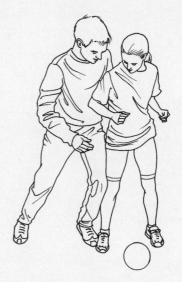

Fortunately, lateral contact injuries rarely require surgery. Since the force from a lateral blow travels across the knee, the most commonly injured structure is the MCL. Unlike the ACL, which tends to rupture when injured, the MCL's injuries are most often sprains (partial tears of the ligament). Sprains are graded I, II, or III, depending on severity. Generally, grade I sprains take four weeks to heal, grade II sprains take six weeks, and grade III sprains take longer than two months. Most MCL injuries are grade I or II, heal without surgery, and allow athletes to return to activity in four to six weeks.

Most Common Injury from Lateral Contact
Medial Collateral Ligament sprain — Grade I
Prognosis: Excellent; most injuries heal within five weeks.

Medial Contact Injuries

Laura, a sixteen-year-old soccer player, was dribbling the ball down the field when another player crashed into the inside of her knee (see Figure 39). Although she was struck from the inside of her knee,

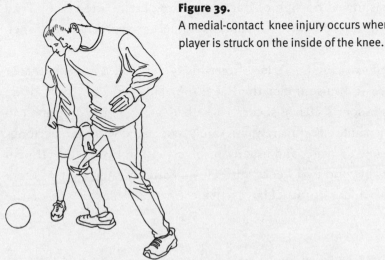

Figure 39.
A medial-contact knee injury occurs when a player is struck on the inside of the knee.

she felt a sharp pain on the outside. The knee did not swell. When I examined Laura's knee in my office, the most notable symptom was the pain along the outside part of the knee in the area of the lateral collateral ligament.

The lateral collateral ligament (LCL) is the structure most usually injured by medial contact, that is, force exerted on the inside of the knee. LCL injuries are usually sprains and heal within three to five weeks. These are usually more serious than MCL injuries and should always be seen by a doctor.

> ## Most Common Injury from Medial Contact
> Lateral Collateral Ligament sprain — Grade I
> Prognosis: Good; most injuries heal within five to six weeks.

Patellar Contusion

A hockey player, tripped from behind, fell hard and directly on his patella (kneecap). He did not twist his knee; the knee did not swell.

X-rays showed no sign of fracture of the patella. He came to my office the next day with pain under his kneecap that was worse when he bent his knee.

The most common injury from this type of fall is called a *patellar contusion* (a bruise under the kneecap). This type of injury often occurs in sports such as soccer, basketball, and rollerblading and can be very painful. Fortunately, it is rarely associated with serious, long-term knee damage, and usually resolves within two weeks. If pain persists beyond two weeks, further evaluation is indicated, as there may be injury to articular cartilage on the undersurface of the patella.

Most Common Injury from Falling Directly on the Patella (Kneecap)

Patellar Contusion
  Prognosis: Excellent; most contusions heal within two weeks.

Prevention of Direct-Contact Injuries

PATIENT: "Hey, doc, it hurts when I do this."

DOCTOR: "So don't do it."

This time-honored exchange certainly applies to contact knee injuries. The best way to prevent them is, obviously, to avoid contact. But in sports such as hockey and football, contact is not only unavoidable but essential, so the only effective prevention strategy is to protect the patellae. Kneepads that are hard on the front and soft on the back are manufactured specifically for rollerblading, hockey, and football. Use the protective gear! I recommend purchasing these pads for each child. Though this can be costly, I see many patellar injuries that result from either a lack of protection ("I didn't wear my kneepads") or from a child's wearing hand-me-down kneepads that don't fit. Remember, kneepads are sized to fit within a few centimeters. It is wise to buy the right size.

Some hockey leagues keep protective gear in a collective pool. The kids use the proper-size gear and then return it for other children to use the following year.

Knee Pain in the Absence of Injury

Stephen, a sixteen-year-old cross-country runner, came to my office complaining of pain in the front of his knee, especially after he climbed stairs or sat for prolonged periods of time. He couldn't remember a specific injury: no falls, no twists, nothing. He described the pain as under the patella. Stephen's knee exam was basically normal — there was no swelling — except that his knee hurt when he bent it and especially when he went up and down stairs. I diagnosed patellofemoral knee pain, otherwise known as a painful kneecap.

Even in the absence of knee injury, young athletes often complain of knee pain: "My knee hurts when I run"; "My knee hurts when I go up and down stairs." Parents are then faced with the difficult task of trying to figure out when a knee injury is serious enough to see a doctor.

Keys to Recognizing Patellofemoral Knee Pain

- Worse with knee bends (up and down stairs).
- Knee rarely swells.
- Pain relieved by ice for fifteen minutes.
- Worst pain occurs during growth years.

Treatment

Ice versus Heat

Parents often ask about using ice and heat for relief of patellofemoral pain. A good rule is to heat the knee for fifteen minutes prior to any athletic activity, using a hot shower or a heating pad. After exercise, it's important to ice down the knee for fifteen minutes. This helps control swelling underneath the kneecap. Frozen peas make the best ice bag because they mold to the knee, hold the molded shape, and run little risk of being eaten by hungry family members.

Knee Brace

Another common treatment of patellofemoral knee pain is using a neoprene knee brace, which works like a scuba suit, trapping body heat and elevating the temperature around the knee. With patellofemoral pain, the kneecap feels better during exercise when the temperature is raised. That is why children with this problem feel better after a hot shower. I suggest a brace with a hole in the center called a patellar buttress brace. For short-term use, I have no problem with the knee brace. In general, however, I dislike the long-term use of knee braces in young athletes because kids can become brace-dependent.

In almost every case, a stretching and strengthening program, as detailed below, is an effective way to treat and prevent patellofemoral pain. If athletes rely too much on the brace, they tend to be unenthusiastic about using a stretching and strengthening program to keep this problem from recurring.

Prevention of Patellofemoral Knee Pain

With knee pain in the absence of knee injury, flexibility is of tremendous importance. The patella is a sesamoid bone, a bone that sits inside a muscle–tendon group. Therefore, the force exerted on the patella is directly proportional to the force exerted by the quad and hamstring muscles. Since kids' bones grow before their muscles do, they actually lose flexibility as they grow (an eight-year-old can much more easily bend over and touch his toes than a fourteen-year-old can). The progressive loss of flexibility, particularly in the muscles around the knee, is a main reason why patellofemoral knee pain is primarily a teenage problem, and also why any athlete or child complaining of knee pain must work on stretching exercises.

Muscle strength can also be a factor. Patellofemoral pain can result from muscle imbalance. Most often, the imbalance arises because the strength in the outside part of the quadriceps muscles (the vastus lateralis) is much stronger than the inside portion (the vastus medialis). Sports entailing a lot of running tend to build up the outside leg muscles. Even in young athletes with very strong leg muscles, such as soccer and tennis players, a strength imbalance can exist between the muscles around the kneecap.

Sometimes a strengthening program is used in conjunction with a stretching program to address muscle imbalance. As the muscles around the patella become more flexible and equally balanced, the force displaced over the anterior portion of the knee is decreased. Muscle groups to emphasize include the hamstring, quadriceps, and hip flexor muscles. This type of stretching and strengthening program is easily obtained from the athletic trainer who works with many school-sponsored sports teams; start looking for information by consulting the athletic trainer.

I encourage young athletes with patellofemoral pain to follow this type of strengthening program for six weeks. It is often helpful to ask an athletic trainer for more advice about such programs, especially since schools and gyms have different resources. The local trainer will know more about the specific situation in your area. The two exercises pictured in Figures 40 and 41 are designed to stretch and strengthen the quadriceps muscles.

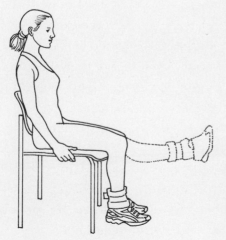

Figure 40.
Quadriceps-strengthening exercise.

Figure 41.
Quadriceps-stretching exercise.

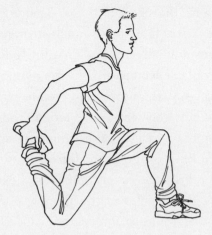

A rule about stretching and strengthening: An adolescent can never stretch, strengthen, or study too much. I encourage all my young patients with patellofemoral knee pain to stretch and strengthen the major leg-muscle groups three times daily. The whole routine takes just fifteen minutes and is very effective; parents and children are always amazed by how well this program works. Don't be discouraged if the results aren't evident in the first few weeks. In general, these programs take four to six weeks to begin showing results.

The Box Score

- Be familiar with common lower-body injuries.
- If a knee or ankle swells, have it evaluated.
- Prevention is key.
- If pain persists for more than 4 weeks, have the knee or ankle evaluated by a doctor.

Common Knee Injuries

	ACL rupture	MCL sprain	Patellar contusion	Meniscus tear	Patello-femoral pain
Mechanism of injury	Twisting, noncontact injury	Struck on the outside of the knee	Fall directly onto kneecap	Twisting, noncontact injury	No specific mechanism for injury; pain with bending
Swelling?	Yes, usually within 1 hour of injury	Rarely	Rarely	Usually	Almost never
"Pop"?	Almost always	Sometimes, with grade II or III injuries	Never	Usually	Never
Able to run after injury?	Knee feels "loose," problem with side-to-side running	Rarely	Depends on severity of injury	Depends on severity of tear	Yes, children can run around with this
Will it require surgery?	Yes, this ligament doesn't heal without surgery	Almost never	Never	Usually, though some small tears can heal in children	Never; treatment through increasing quadriceps strength and flexibility

Chapter 11

Pigskin and Sheepskin

THINKING ABOUT COLLEGE

*This chapter suggests questions to ask about playing sports in college
and describes the recruitment process.*

When their child stars on his high school varsity team, many
parents envision a free ride at a top college. And beyond
college lie the dazzling million-dollar contracts of the
NBA, NFL, or MLB.

Face facts, folks: With very few exceptions, it's not going to happen. The NCAA (National Collegiate Athletic Association) points
out that every year about 1 million high school boys play football
and 550,000 play basketball. The number of college football players
per year is 56,000, the number of male college basketball players
about 16,000. These college numbers include players who suit up
but never play, not to mention players on the practice squad who
never even suit up. In other words, a high school football player has
less than a 6 in 100 chance of making a college team, a high school
basketball player less than a 3 in 100 chance. Furthermore, these
numbers include roster spots at colleges that do not offer athletic
scholarships at all. The chances of a high school athlete's ever making it to the pros are, obviously, far smaller. The NCAA says a high

school senior playing football has less than a 1 in 1,000 chance of ever being drafted by a professional team, a high school senior basketball player less than a 3 in 10,000 chance! So much for hoop dreams.

So the likelihood of a high school player's making a college varsity team is extremely small, and of winning an athletic scholarship even smaller.

Except for the tiny number of players who will benefit from showcasing their talent there for the pro scouts, the primary reason for an athlete to go to college is to get an education, which is only becoming more important as society advances technologically. Even for the handful of athletes who become pros, their careers are short (unless they're golfers) and they still need to find meaningful work, which is a lot easier to do with an educated mind. It is also true that for some students, the only way to pay for college is through athletics, but those very students are frequently short-changed educationally. At many colleges they are segregated from the general student body, spending most of their waking hours working out or traveling for the team, taking courses and majors especially designed for athletes.

For every student, choosing a college should be done with great care. The choice is not just about the next four years, but about a lifetime of friends, acquaintances, and advisers, about values manifested by the school and embraced by the student. It's about finding a place where the student will broaden not only her intellectual world, but her social one, as she gets to know people from different backgrounds.

In the case of the athlete, the question of fit is twofold. He must feel comfortable with the program, the team, and the coach, which means he thinks he has something to offer and that he will learn and grow from them in return. He must also feel comfortable with the world of the college. If in order to play on a team he likes, he chooses a college well below his intellectual gifts — a college where, say, his older teammates turn to him, a freshman, as the resident genius who can help them with their papers — his classes are likely to be geared to a lower level than he will find stimulating, and he will feel academically and socially isolated. On the other hand, if he attends an academically prestigious school where students eagerly pursue philosophical discussions at all hours of the night, he may well find himself isolated there as well, and worse, assumed to be a lunkhead by both peers and professors.

The admissions numbers at high-profile colleges doom most to disappointment. The admissions process is complicated and stressful. Parents and students alike feel their lives are being judged by unfeeling outsiders, and unfortunately they are more or less correct. College admissions all too often feel like the great final report card that grades parenthood. It is important to recognize that many excellent colleges exist, and that the goal is for the student to find a place where he can thrive, where he is comfortable, and where he is challenged but not overwhelmed.

And even if your student isn't interested in continuing her sport in college, having been committed to sports, whether playing on the varsity team or coaching youth soccer, is one kind of experience that develops character and leadership. Colleges want active, interesting individuals who have demonstrated leadership and contribute to their community.

The prospective college athlete and his parents should ask themselves:

- Does the student want to play in college?
- Is the student good enough to play in college?

Only if both questions are answered yes should a parent think about the next two questions, which overlap a lot:

- Is she good enough to be recruited?
- Is she good enough to get an athletic scholarship?

And if these are answered yes, then perhaps parents should think about ways to help their child get noticed by coaches. But first consider what these questions mean.

Playing in College

Does your student want to play in college?

What does playing in college entail? In many colleges, sports encompass a great variety of competition, from novice to near-pro, from club or intramural teams to junior varsity and varsity teams. A student may want to continue playing, but not with the commitment required for varsity. For this student, JV, intramural, or house teams are an excellent opportunity.

College varsity athletics differ from high school primarily in their intensity and the greater amount of time demanded of the player. The travel time alone, to conference and nonconference games, is considerable.

The level of varsity competition differs significantly among the various types of colleges. Most colleges belong to an intercollegiate athletic association that organizes and administers all areas of extramural sports. The NCAA is the largest of these. Others include the NAIA (National Association of Intercollegiate Athletics) and the NJCAA (National Junior College Athletic Association). The NCAA's Divisions I, II, and III are categorized by the amount of resources dedicated to athletics, or, basically, the number of sports a school sponsors, and whether and how much money is awarded as scholarships for athletic ability.

The NCAA governs four major areas of athletics: playing and practice season; financial aid; recruiting practices; and eligibility (which in Division III is determined by each institution but in Division I is regulated by the NCAA). The rules are many and complicated. Some are as specific as the number of contacts allowed from college coach to player, the number of the player's paid visits to the college, the number of scholarships, how scholarships are divided. Some, especially the rules regarding academic eligibility, change periodically. At this time, to be eligible for a college athletic scholarship, the student must graduate from high school after successfully completing thirteen core academic courses, maintaining a 2.5 GPA, and scoring a combined minimum of 820 on the math and verbal SATs. To play on Division I or II teams, a student must have his academic eligibility certified by the NCAA Initial Eligibility Clearinghouse. More detailed information about NCAA rules is available on their website, www.ncaa.org. The other associations have similar sets of rules.

NCAA Division I, II, and III Membership Criteria

Division I member institutions have to sponsor at least seven sports for men and seven for women (or six for men and eight for women) with two team sports for each gender. Each playing season has to be represented by each gender as well (fall, winter, spring). There are contest and participant minimums for each sport, as well as scheduling criteria. For sports other than football and basketball, Div. I schools must play 100% of the minimum number of contests against Div. I opponents — anything over the minimum number of games has to be 50% Div. I. Men's and women's basketball teams have to play all but two games against Div. I teams; for men, they must play ⅓ of all their contests in the home arena. Schools that have football are classified as Div. I-A or I-AA. I-A football schools are usually fairly elaborate programs. Div. I-A teams have to meet minimum attendance requirements (17,000 people in attendance per home game, OR 20,000 average of all football games in the last four years, or 30,000 permanent seats in their stadium and average 17,000 per home game or 20,000 average of all football games in the last four years, OR be in a member conference in which at least six conference members sponsor football or more than half of football schools meet attendance criteria. Div. I-AA teams do not need to meet minimum attendance requirements. Div. I schools must meet minimum financial aid awards for their athletics program, and there are maximum financial aid awards for each sport that a Div. I school cannot exceed.

Division II institutions have to sponsor at least four sports for men and four for women, with two team sports for each gender, and each playing season represented by each gender. There are contest and participant minimums for each sport, as well as scheduling criteria — football and men's and women's basketball teams must play at least 50% of their games against Div. II or I-A or I-AA opponents. For sports other than football and basketball there are no scheduling requirements. There are not attendance requirements for football, or arena game requirements for basketball. There are maximum financial aid awards for each sport that a Div. II school must not exceed.

Division III institutions have to sponsor at least five sports for men and five for women, with two team sports for each gender, and each playing season represented by each gender. There are minimum contest and participant minimums for each sport. Division III athletics features student-athletes who receive no financial aid related to their athletic ability and athletic departments are staffed and funded like any other department in the university. Division III athletics departments place special importance on the impact of athletics on the participants rather than on the spectators. . . . Division III athletics encourages participation by maximizing the number and variety of athletics opportunities available to students . . .

Source: http://ncaa.org/about/div_criteria.html

The NCAA divisions are important for kids considering playing in college because they reflect the level of competition, determine the number of hours — and months — that can be required of a student athlete, and govern whether or not a college can offer athletic scholarships. Division I colleges offer the most competitive, visible athletics, Division III the least. Division I offers athletic scholarships, Division III does not. (*Note:* In Division I football, schools are either I-A or I-AA, the distinction being the size of the program and the number of athletic scholarships they offer. Ivy League schools are Division I-AA and do not offer athletic scholarships.) Division I colleges can range from highly selective academic institutions (Stanford, Princeton), to large state universities known for excellence in both academics and athletics (Michigan, UCLA), to state schools whose renown rests in large part on athletics (University of Nevada–Las Vegas, University of Nebraska). Division III generally means smaller liberal arts colleges (such as Haverford, Williams, Colgate, Macalester); some Division III schools are much more committed to athletics than others are, and some Division III schools focus their resources on a few selected sports. Division II colleges lie in between and tend to be large — 7,000 to 8,000 students (University of Bridgeport, University of California–Davis).

In general, college varsity sports differ from high school in that they demand greater speed, skill, and contact. If your child is a highly skilled soccer player but dislikes getting hit, Division I may not be for her.

College sports also demand a greater commitment of time. D-I coaches can require twenty hours a week from their athletes three seasons a year. D-III coaches can require twenty hours of practice but only in season. (This means that Division III students can play two or more sports if they choose.) Note, however, that the twenty hours of practice do not include time spent on showers, weight training, watching videotapes. Furthermore, a scheduled competition counts as three hours, even if players have to fly cross-country to get there. In addition, many coaches require, or highly recommend, summer training programs. All expect their players to show up at school in peak physical fitness.

Going to college means getting a formal education, but it can also mean exposure to a wider expanse of interests and activities. Is the student willing to forgo this opportunity to stretch? While being on a college team offers an established community of interest, that community can also be constricting. Is the student willing and temperamentally suited to make the extra effort to meet different kinds of students? Is he willing to sacrifice time spent hanging with friends, dating, meeting and arguing with people who have different ideas about how the world works or what's important in life? Is he willing to spend his summers keeping himself in peak physical condition?

Making the Cut

Is your student good enough to play in college?

A kid may be a star athlete at his high school, but the United States is a big country. How does he stack up against other high school stars coast to coast and, these days, from foreign countries as well? Is he in an Olympic Development Program, being recommended or recruited for regional and state teams? It's not uncommon for a star high school pitcher to end up riding the bench, or not making the team, at Division I schools that are hardly known as incubators of Major League talent. The level of the specific team also makes a difference. A water polo patient of mine was admitted to two Division I athletic powerhouses; she knew by comparing her skill level to older hometown teammates' at these schools that if she went to the West Coast she wouldn't make the team, whereas at the East Coast school she would start. She chose the East. I'm not naming names because I don't want to incur the wrath of any admissions departments at schools where I might want to send my offspring. I'm also not naming names because standings change — some years College X is great at women's tennis, other years the talent goes elsewhere.

In general, however, a student hoping to play for a Division I team should be an all-state, all-regional, or national player or champion and should train or cross-train all year round. Division II teams are less rigorous but are still looking for regional-level players. Division III teams are looking for excellent high school athletes. As mentioned above, however, even schools within the same division vary widely in their commitment to sports. A further wrinkle is that some

D-III programs are more competitive than some D-I programs. When starting to think about college, however, students and parents should keep the basic generalizations in mind.

Here are some questions to help student and parents assess athletic performance.

What level does she play at: school only? club? regional? national? How does she compare to others in her sport? What honors or awards has she received? What are her statistics (times, goals scored, and so on)? These vary, of course, by sport, and are more difficult to define and compile for team players than those in individual sports, and more difficult still for defensive players than offensive players. (Defensive stats can include number of blocks and rebounds in basketball; clearances, tackles, and percentage of tackles won in soccer.)

What is his foot speed? Reaction time when receiving the ball, whether a soccer ball or a baseball? Speed and soundness of his decision-making? How productive are his decisions?

If you or your child cannot answer these questions, he's probably not a D-I candidate.

Is the athlete willing to sit on the bench, and for how long? College teams need to maintain a certain GPA as a whole and will sometimes take an excellent student to raise that average. If your child just wants to be on a team, being a bench player or on the practice squad is one way to achieve that objective.

To assess a student's performance, ask for a candid opinion from his own coach and opposing coaches as well. Good coaches make it their business to check out the local, if not regional, talent pool, and most are pleased to offer their evaluation of a player's skills and talents. Also be sure to ask the coaches and faculty at summer sports camps for an evaluation; camp staff expect to be asked. In addition, most college coaches issue a candidate questionnaire that helps players quantify information about the level of skills and competitiveness of team(s) played on.

When looking at colleges and teams, keep in mind that different coaches value different abilities and characteristics. They have different coaching styles (some want more control, some want more creativity from players). When a coach is filling in a roster, he may need just the qualities and skills your child can provide. On the other hand, if your child is an outstanding point guard and the college she prefers already has five, she would do well to look elsewhere.

Recruitment

Is your student good enough to be recruited?

Being recruited means that a college coach is interested in an athlete's being on his team. Recruitment can mean help with admissions and with getting an athletic scholarship.

Most recruiting arises from college coaches talking to their networks of contacts — other coaches in precollege leagues. They ask how an athlete compares to other students in that league, and how the best in that league compare to athletes on a national level. Camps run on college campuses and high-level tournaments, such as those of the AAU (Amateur Athletic Union) and ODP (Olympic Development Program), are also significant recruiting vehicles today. They provide an efficient way for coaches to see many top athletes at the same time, playing against better competition than in high school games.

Recruitment ultimately means being put on the list the coach submits to the admissions office. Each sport has a certain number of slots available, the list is longer than the number of slots, and the coach ranks kids in order of desirability (the ones at the top are the best athletes, those at the bottom may or may not have slightly better grades). Coaches are interested in three factors when listing a student: intent to come, athletic ability, and academic status. No prospect can be a zero in any one factor, but to a coach, intent to come and athletic ability far outweigh academic standing.

The power of the coach's list is different at different colleges and obviously depends on how important sports are and how important the particular team is at the school. At some schools, the coach's picks — especially in the so-called revenue sports of football and basketball — are virtually guaranteed admission (although candidates must meet the NCAA criteria). At other schools, even if the coach designates someone as a must-have, the admissions office has the final say in the decision.

Thus, being told one is "on the list" does not mean automatic admission. Even at schools where the football coach is paid more than the college president, being high on the list is better than being toward the bottom but still guarantees nothing. Students and their families should also remember that just as they should be pressing more than one college, keeping their options open, seeking the best opportunities, coaches know that many colleges are talking to the same athletes. Recruitment is a two-way process. Coaches are looking for the best candidates they can find and talking to more students than they have room for on their list. Some coaches are overly optimistic about their clout with the admissions office; a few are consciously manipulative and misrepresent what they will do for a prospect. So even if the college coach is very enthusiastic and attentive, admission is official only when the letter comes from the college admissions office.

The NCAA and other associations have strict rules about the number of calls a Division I coach can make and when; how many paid visits an athlete can make to a college and for how long; what expenses are legitimate and what aren't. Basically, contact from the coaching staff and alumni, whether in person or by phone, is strictly limited by recruiting regulations and cannot take place until July 1 after the student's junior year in high school. You might hear or read about a star athlete's being offered a full university scholarship in his junior year of high school. Keep in mind the following: Journalists love flashy stories; families of athletes can be as competitive as the athletes themselves and might misunderstand or distort the facts; the NCAA does not allow contact with or a scholarship offer to a high school junior, and coaches and colleges comply with these rules. *Note:* A Division I coach is not allowed even to return a phone call until July 1 of an athlete's junior year.

At the very top level of recruited students are the "blue chip" athletes, the national record holders or state champions, the obvious stars. The local television station shows up for their events and recruiters have circled them since early in their careers. These chosen few already know who they are, they have their choice of colleges, and their parents probably aren't reading this chapter.

Next in the hierarchy are the regional and state players, the ones who attend summer sports camp and have attracted attention from the faculty and staff coaches. As in any profession, there are informal networks of coaches who talk to each other about the available and upcoming talent. Much recruitment at this level takes place here.

Athletic programs at D-II and III colleges are lower-profile than those of D-I schools, but their academic and athletic offerings can be completely satisfying to students, and the level of pressure and competition may be more suitable. Kids who want to play or who need financial support should not rule out these schools, which also recruit athletes for their teams. Although Division I offers the most athletic scholarships per sport, Division II also offers athletic scholarships, and Division III offers financial aid.

Nonrecruited athletes who try out in college are called *walk-ons*, and they often must demonstrate skills and heart beyond not only those of their fellow freshmen, but of the team veterans. On the day that walk-ons are allowed to show up, the coach often makes practice unusually grueling. It is possible for walk-ons to earn an athletic scholarship if the coach finds them sufficiently productive, but those who make the team are more likely to be bench players or on the scout team. This was the case of Rudy Ruettiger, whose story of making the Notre Dame football practice squad is depicted in the movie *Rudy*. There are, however, rare and great exceptions, such as Steve Shak, who walked on to play soccer for UCLA, helped them win the 1997 NCAA title, and was the number-one draft pick for Major League Soccer's MetroStars.

Getting in the Recruitment Game

If your child wants to play in college, he should make sure to get himself into the recruiting process. (Coaches promise many things — playing time, positions, scholarship money — to recruited athletes; they have little left to offer to someone they've never seen before.) This is particularly important in the D-I schools, where virtually all varsity players are recruited, but it is also important for the other NCAA divisions; in D-III, depending on the school and the sport, perhaps half the varsity players have not been recruited out of high school. This number seems to be growing smaller, however, as Division III schools recruit more and more of their athletes.

The NCAA sponsors twenty-two championship sports, and about 353,400 young men and women play college varsity sports. Very few high school students enjoy the privilege of sitting back and being sought out by college coaches. Most need to work to get recruited. The task is enormous and demands great initiative, organization, and skill at negotiation (especially if scholarships are involved). Parents need to be active in helping their children through this process.

If your child is hoping to be recruited, start planning early (sophomore year of high school is typical). The following outlines what she must do, with your help, in addition to the general college application process.

- Keep a résumé of stats, achievements, and awards; save any newspaper clippings that mention her.
- Play on the most competitive teams she can and go to high-visibility tournaments where college coaches are in attendance. (Parents should consider the time and expense in relation to the needs of the rest of the family. They might deem the time and money needed for this kind of participation a good investment, but if the child does not win a large scholarship, will they feel like failures and blame the child?)

- Attend summer camps where college coaches can see her play, especially after her junior year. (Some camps offer tuition scholarships.)
- Research many suitable colleges, consulting the school guidance counselor and her coaches, and the numerous books available on the subject.
- Initiate contact with the coaches of the teams she's interested in, rather than the athletic directors. Her letters should be clear, free of spelling and grammatical errors, and should give sufficient information about her athletic abilities and why she's interested in the school/coach. She should respond promptly when she hears from coaches at schools she's interested in and write thank-you notes.
- Ask her coaches and college counselors to put in a word for her with college coaches in her sport (not the athletic director) at the schools she wishes to attend.
- Register with the NCAA Initial Eligibility Clearinghouse.
- Produce a videotape that identifies who she is and shows highlights of her play in several games or one whole game. (Some coaches want to see a long segment of a game, some prefer highlights. Find out ahead of time what a particular coach wants to see before sending a tape.) Some high schools can help with videotaping — ask the coach.
- Study the NCAA's or other association's rules. If your child breaks the rules, however inadvertently, she will be unable to play.
- Ask the college coach questions, to help your child decide what school to attend.
- Be candid and enthusiastic, keep many irons in the fire, and remember that acceptance is not official until the letter comes from the college admissions office.

Most students visit colleges at their own expense, but if a D-I college is very interested in a particular student, its athletic department is allowed to pay for one forty-eight-hour visit when the student is a senior. Students must also prepare for being interviewed by the coach: They should be able to cite their statistics and describe their abilities, but not sound too arrogant or too humble. They should also be honest about their needs and intentions. Don't let your child distort the facts. (I believe parents should be concerned first and foremost with their child's character. But also, to be very practical, the world of coaching is very small. The coaches generally know each other, especially those in the same conference, and they talk.)

Athletic Scholarships

Colleges help families pay the high costs of tuition in two ways. They offer *financial aid*, which is awarded on the basis of demonstrated need. Financial aid is usually a package of grants, low-interest loans, and a work-study job. The other way to get help with the costs is through *merit scholarships*, which are awarded for academic, artistic, and athletic excellence, regardless of need.

Division I and II colleges offer full and partial athletic scholarships, granted one year at a time. If an athlete is injured, or decides he no longer wants to play (for example, he's burnt out, he can't keep up with his studies, he finds the coach incompetent or abusive), or his grades make him ineligible, the scholarship can be revoked. In contrast, financial aid is canceled only if a student drops out of school.

It's difficult to make a Division I team. It's even more difficult to get a scholarship to do so. The student must be a top-level athlete, have acceptable grades and SAT scores, and persuade the coach that he is necessary enough to the team to be granted one of the school's limited number of athletic scholarships. The better the grades, the easier it will be for a coach to award him tuition money. Consider the following numbers: In Division I-A football, schools are allowed to offer a maximum of 85 athletic scholarships but the average

I-A squad is 113.9 students. In Division I women's gymnastics, schools can offer a maximum of 12 scholarships, but the average squad is 16.7.

The situation is even more complicated than these numbers suggest because money can be awarded as full or partial scholarships.

The kids offered the limited number of full athletic scholarships are the kids seen at summer sports camps with college coaches as faculty; some play football or basketball in big public high schools where recruiters are looking for them; some play in high-profile clubs or tournaments where the coaches discuss big talent with college coaches they know. Some are seen by alumni, who call in reports to the athletic department. The chosen student signs a letter of intent, committing herself to attend that college, and the admissions process occurs much sooner than for other students. When a coach offers an athletic scholarship, he has usually already checked with the admissions department to be sure the student is admissible, so the scholarship offer generally means automatic admission. The student, however, must still meet the NCAA minimum academic requirements and keep her grades up while at college.

Pros and Cons

Athletic scholarships are rare, and they are not a free ride. The demands they put on the student's time are severe. Athletic scholarships do not have to be paid back, but they can be awarded only one year at a time. (If a four-year free ride is offered, it's illegal recruiting.) And if the student is injured or takes a semester off to study, the scholarship is likely to be rescinded. On the other hand, if the student's family is wealthy, he is still eligible for an athletic scholarship and his parents can spend the projected tuition money to buy him a car or set up a trust fund.

Some 150,000 college athletic scholarships (full and partial) are offered each year in more than thirty sports, from football to golf to downhill skiing. Many more academic scholarships are available (some estimate ten times as many), which are awarded based on academic achievement.

Only Division I and II schools offer athletic scholarships. The Ivy League schools offer none (although they might make it easy for a desired athlete to pay his tuition by offering liberal financial aid or undemanding work-study jobs). Division III schools offer no athletic scholarships, but those that consider sports important can offer generous financial aid to athletes they consider desirable.

Choosing a College

After narrowing down the list of colleges, the student athlete should find out more about the programs before deciding where to go. Here are some questions to ask the prospective college coach:

- How much time practice time is scheduled?
- How much additional training time is expected? During the season? Out of season?
- How long is the season?
- How often and how far does the team regularly travel?
- How many games are scheduled per season?
- What services are available for athletes: health, training, and rehabilitation facilities? meals? housing? tutoring?
- What circumstances would cause an athletic scholarship to be withdrawn? What happens in the case of injury?
- What positions/events is the student being considered for?
- What do the coaches do to integrate the athletes into the general student body?

While visiting a college she's interested in, the student should see a game to learn more about the coach's philosophy, approach to the players, and behavior in general. What does the coach value? Does he want to win no matter what? (The visiting student should try to ask players how the coach behaves after a win, a loss.) Would it be fun to play for this coach? What will the student learn from this coach?

The Box Score

- The odds of playing Division I are minuscule, of getting a scholarship even smaller.
- The purpose of attending college is intellectual, emotional, and social growth.
- When deciding on a college, try to keep an honest perspective on what your child wants to do in life beyond college.
- Grades — in high school *and* in college — are important.
- Financial aid is based on demonstrated family need. Scholarships are need-blind and awarded for merit, usually academic, artistic, or athletic.
- Playing college sports should be fun. Will playing enhance the college experience? Is playing the only way to pay the tuition?
- Getting recruited takes work.

Notes from the Doctor

Photocopy the following pages and keep them in your child's or coach's sports bag for when you cannot consult a doctor face to face.

Concussion

Concussions (also known as closed head injuries) are high-contact injuries to the brain. They are very common in high-contact sports such as football, soccer, and rugby. The incidence of concussion is estimated at 300,000 per year, making it the most common head injury associated with sports participation.

If you have a football player, the helmet needs to fit properly to minimize concussion risk, as is the case with biking and rollerblading.

Not all concussions are the same. They are graded, and the response to each grade is different.

The signs and proper treatment of concussion are important for parents, coaches, and players to know. The key to healthy sports participation is good prevention and appropriate response to significant injuries. An athlete should never return to competition after a concussion without first being cleared by a health professional.

Grade	Symptoms	What to Do
Grade I — the most common	Player has dazed look, talks of having his "bell rung"; is dizzy for some time after initial injury; and suffers some memory loss.	Get player off the field. He can return to the game if he can run on the sideline with no symptoms of headache or dizziness.
Grade II	Loss of consciousness for less than 5 minutes, a "blackout."	Remove player from competition and stop all participation in contact sports until the player's physician has given clearance to play.
Grade III	Loss of consciousness for more than 5 minutes.	Take player directly to the emergency room, even if he wakes up and looks normal.

Heading the Soccer Ball: A Cause for Concern?

Parents, coaches, and players often ask whether repeatedly heading the soccer ball can cause brain injury. Most of the medical studies that address this issue seem to indicate that hitting the ball with one's head is not injurious to the brain or to long-term cognitive function.

What might have some longer-term effects, however, is repeated concussions as a child or teen. These injuries, even at grade I level, have been shown to cause changes on tests of cognition and mental functioning. The best response is to prevent them from happening.

For soccer, this means making sure that the ball size is correct for the age of the athlete, and that kids avoid jumping into each other when heading and that they play by the rules. Proper heading technique is also important, starting from the back, with a rigid neck pushing through the ball.

Guidelines for Hydration:
Before, During, and After Sports

- Proper hydration can improve performance and diminish fatigue and can actually reduce the chance of muscle injury (strain).
- Hydration is especially important when the temperature is over 70 degrees.
- Starting children with effective hydration techniques when they are young encourages effective hydration behavior throughout their sports career.

12–24 hours before event	During event	8 hours after event
Drink enough water so that the urine is almost colorless.	Drink ½ cup to 1 cup (4 to 8 ounces) of water or sports drink every 15 to 20 minutes depending on tolerance (not juice or carbonated soda — they have too much carbohydrate for easy absorption).	Drink 2 to 4 cups (16 to 24 ounces) for each pound of weight lost during exercise.

Note: An athlete does not need to feel thirsty to be dehydrated.

When to Go to the Emergency Room

- Stay calm. Panic only makes the situation worse.
- Don't move anyone who is lying on the field hurt; wait for medical help to arrive.
- Is there a doctor in the house? Find out whether a health professional is nearby.

- Significant swelling (compared to the corresponding area on the other side of the body) generally means the injury is more serious and needs attention.
- Bluish skin often means bleeding underneath, which means the injury might be more serious.
- Athletes younger than twelve have a higher index of suspicion for injury, since the growth plates are open.

Notes on the Emergency Room

In general, many more injured athletes go to the emergency room than is absolutely necessary. An alternative to the emergency room is RICE (rest, ice, compression, elevation) and seeing a physician the next day.

Take to Emergency Room Today	Take to Doctor Tomorrow
Dislocated joint (finger, shoulder)	Sprained ankle
Pain in wrist after a fall	Bruise
Limping child under age 12 who has swelling or pain in the ankle or foot	Injuries without significant swelling
Concussion followed by loss of consciousness	Injuries where players can continue to play despite the pain
Tooth knocked out of mouth — clean the tooth and put it back in its socket, or better yet, have the player put it under his tongue and see a doctor the same day.	

RICE: For sprains, strains, swellings, and other aches and pains

RICE is the acronym for Rest, Ice, Compression, and Elevation. Employ RICE during the first twenty-four to forty-eight hours after injury.

- Rest. That is, keep the involved area still for one or two days. Rest is the most important component of RICE.
- Ice. Ice will diminish swelling and help control the pain. Apply ice to the injured area for fifteen to twenty minutes every hour. Prompt ice treatment speeds healing by 50 percent, allowing a patient to resume activity more quickly.
- Compression. An Ace wrap to apply gentle compression to the area will help reduce swelling. Don't wrap the bandage too tightly — just enough to supply a gentle squeeze.
- Elevation. Position the injured limb on a pillow to raise it above the level of the heart. This will help reduce swelling.

Note 1: Children with open growth plates (generally, girls under age twelve and boys under age fourteen) should have injuries to arms, legs, and shoulders evaluated by a physician.

Note 2: If the skin develops a bluish color or the pain is not reduced within twenty-four hours, consult a physician.

After thirty-six to forty-eight hours, after swelling goes down, apply heat to increase blood flow and bring more oxygen and nutrients to aid healing.

Playing Through the Pain

This classic phrase is often used in such sports as football, running, and ballet to describe the ideal, heroic behavior of the true athlete. Parents should know, however, that playing through the pain is a bad idea, especially for kids. Kids' bodies are still developing, and their bones have open growth plates. When kids play through the pain, they can aggravate injuries such as stress fractures or develop problems such as Little League shoulder that lead to problems with bone growth later in life.

As a general rule, then, kids *should not* play through the pain. However —

It's okay to play when the pain:

- Does not interfere with performance.
- Does not cause a limp or other noticeable effect.

It's *not* okay to play when the pain:

- Causes limping or other noticeable effects.
- Interferes with performance.
- Leads a child to not want to play.

See a doctor if there is:

- Swelling.
- Pain for more than three weeks.
- Pain that worsens over time.

What Is a Trainer?

The generic term *trainer* is used widely in sports, but there are several different kinds of trainer. A personal trainer, who earns certification by participating in a weekend training program, works at a gym or in the homes of individuals. Some personal trainers are authoritative sources of information, while others know very little about injury. An athletic trainer (ATC), who is always found on the sideline of professional and collegiate sporting events and increasingly so at the high school and junior high level, is a valuable resource for players and parents but often underutilized. Athletic trainers complete a college degree in sideline medical care. Trained in injury evaluation, they help decide if someone needs to go immediately to the emergency room or can wait until the next day to see a doctor. They are very skilled at taping up ankles, knees, and wrists. I advise parents to make contact with the school or league athletic trainer at the beginning of the playing season to become familiar with what an athletic trainer has to offer. For more information about athletic trainers, see the National Athletic Trainers' Association Web site, www.nata.org.

What to Do in Case Of:

Note: These are general guidelines only for common sports injuries. Whenever possible, consult your own physician.

Back pain. See a doctor if the pain worsens for more than two weeks, if pain at night wakes the child from sleep, if pain in the back radiates to a leg, or if there is any tingling or numbness in a leg or foot. Otherwise, the child can keep playing.

Bruised ribs. If a rib is fractured (broken), it can puncture a lung, which is a serious injury. See a doctor if (a) the ribs hurt with breathing or (b) the pain worsens. If there is shortness of breath, go to the ER. If the pain is localized to one spot and hurts for more than three days, go to a doctor for an X-ray to rule out a fracture.

Concussion. Evaluate the grade of concussion (see page 255). If there is any loss of consciousness (LOC), take the child to the local emergency room. If there is no LOC, you can take your child home but be sure to touch base with your pediatrician. Once at home, watch out for a headache that worsens, vomiting, or double vision. With any of these symptoms, call your doctor and go immediately to the emergency room. The day after a grade I concussion, take your child to see your pediatrician. If your child has had more than three concussions, speak with your pediatrician about a referral to a neurologist.

Elbow pain. Since kids until age fourteen have open growth plates in the elbow, any elbow pain that (a) worsens with throwing, (b) persists for more than three weeks, or (c) limits activity should be evaluated by a physician.

Eye injury. Cover the good eye with one hand and test the vision of the injured eye. Go to the ER if vision is diminished or if there is visible blood in the front or bottom of the eye (hyphema). Consult your pediatrician the same day.

Jammed finger. If the finger looks crooked or twisted, or if your child cannot move it, take her immediately to a doctor or emergency room to see about a dislocation or fracture. If there is swelling or pain in the joint (where the finger bends), you can wait till the next day to see a doctor. At home, ice the finger and splint it with a tongue depressor or a stick to keep the finger straight.

Knee pain. See a doctor if (a) the knee is swollen, (b) the child describes the knee as "giving out" with activity, (c) pain persists for more than three weeks, or (d) a twisting injury to the knee is associated with a "popping" sound. The child can play if the knee pain is moderate and doesn't seem to worsen with activity or over time. Pain under the kneecap is the most common type of knee pain in teenagers; it calls for immediate medical attention.

Mononucleosis. Mono swells the lymph tissues, in particular the tonsils (leading to sore throat) and the spleen, which reaches maximum size one month after the onset of the disease. The major potential complicaiton for athletes is a ruptured spleen, which can result from a sharp blow to the abdomen in high-contact sports (football, soccer, basketball). Consult your doctor to determine when your child can safely return to play. Depending on the severity of the case, the athlete may be out for as little as a few days to as much as a month.

Shinsplints. If the pain is alongside the inside of the shin, try orthotics (arch supports) in the shoes. If the pain worsens, or your child says he is having trouble running, take him to a doctor. If the pain hurts with walking as well as with running, consider seeing a doctor. Often an X-ray and subsequent MRI are used to look for a stress fracture. If the pain goes away with running, the child can play, unless it gets worse over time.

Glossary

AC separation. Also known as "separated shoulder"; occurs when an athlete falls onto the shoulder and the ligaments in the acromio-clavicular joint are torn.

ACL rupture. Complete tearing of the anterior cruciate ligament. The ligament snaps like a rubber band. This injury is at least three to four times more common in females than males.

Adolescent development. The overall process of changing from child to teenager — physically, emotionally, psychologically — which usually occurs between the ages of nine and sixteen.

Anabolic steroids. Synthetically produced testosterone derivates that can be taken orally or injected into muscle to increase baseline strength by increasing the anabolic (muscle-building) effects of testosterone. They can also predispose users to increased risk of liver cancer and other medical problems.

Androstenedione. Nutritional supplement touted by manufacturers as a "safe" alternative to anabolic steroids. This compound is not safe, has not been cleared by the FDA, and can cause premature puberty in kids and teens.

Anterior cruciate ligament (ACL). The main ligament in the knee; the ACL runs inside the intercondylar notch and holds the femur and tibia together when the knee twists. The ACL is the only ligament in the knee that requires surgery to repair.

Anterior talofibular ligament (ATFL). The most commonly sprained ligament in the body; located on the outside (lateral) part of the ankle.

Articular cartilage. The cartilage covering the bones in the joints, such as the knee. When the articular cartilage surface wears down, doctors call it osteoarthritis, which is usually what people refer to when they say they have arthritis.

Avulsion fracture. A fracture where a tendon pulls off a piece of bone, usually at the site of a cartilage growth plate.

Axial load injury. Injury resulting from the athlete's landing directly on the shoulder from the side; same mechanism as a clavicle fracture, so with this type of injury the doctor must check for clavicle fracture.

Biomechanics. How someone is built as related to sports. The most common biomechanical problem is pronation, or "rolling in," of the feet, which predisposes an athlete to stress fractures in the feet, legs, and hips. Players can retrain muscles with faulty movement patterns to move efficiently and effectively.

Carbohydrates. One of the three energy-producing nutrients (along with protein and fat), carbohydrates are either complex or simple. **Complex carbohydrates** are starchy carbohydrates found primarily in plants and consumed as cereals, breads, other whole grains, and potatoes. **Simple carbohydrates** are sugars, such as candy, sugared cereal, and just plain sugar.

Cardiovascular conditioning. Heart and lung conditioning. Getting in shape for the season means exercising your heart and lungs to increase their capacity.

Clavicle (collarbone) fracture. Most commonly broken bone in the body; generally occurs when a player lands directly on the shoulder from the side; this is the same mechanism as an axial load injury.

Creatine. Nutritional supplement taken by athletes to improve strength. Not recommended for children and adolescents due to absence of testing in this age group.

Deltoid ligament. Thickest ligament in the ankle; located on inside (medial) of ankle. Injuring this ligament requires significant force.

Discogenic back pain. Back pain due to a bulging disc in the spine; often worsens with bending forward.

Dislocation. When a joint comes fully out of the socket and needs to be put back into place. This is often treated with surgery, especially if there has been more than one episode.

Diuretic. Drug causing rapid weight reduction through loss of water. Prescribed for patients with heart disease, it has also been abused by wrestlers to rapidly reduce weight.

Eversion. Rolling outward on ankle; less common than inversion, but more serious when it occurs.

Exercise-induced asthma (EIA). Shortness of breath and wheezing during and just after intense physical activity. It is not the same as asthma (the actual medical term is *exercise-induced bronchospasm*), and it is present in 95 percent of asthmatics and roughly 15 to 20 percent of the nonasthmatic population.

Fat. One of the three energy-producing nutrients; the body needs very little fat as a nutrient and stores it for long-term energy.

Female athlete triad. Three concurrent unhealthy conditions — anorexia (disordered eating), amenorrhea (absence of menstrual periods), and osteoporosis (low bone density) — that occur in some athletic females.

Glenohumeral dislocation. When the shoulder joint comes fully out of the socket and needs to be put back into place.

Glenohumeral ligament. Ligament that holds the glenohumeral joint in the shoulder together.

Glenohumeral subluxation. Slipping of the main joint in the shoulder (the glenohumeral joint). The joint does not come out of the socket, but slips back into place.

Glucose. The sugar that carbohydrates break down into. It is readily absorbed into the bloodstream.

Glycogen. Stored form of glucose, found mostly in the liver but also in muscle. Glycogen is broken down into glucose for use during exercise.

Growth plate. Found at the ends of most bones in a child and developing teen; made of cartilage, it is prone to injury because it is much softer than bone.

Intercondylar notch. Space where cruciate ligaments in the knee are located.

Inversion. Classic type of rolling over, or rolling inward, on the ankle.

Lateral. Outside.

Ligament. Connective tissue that ties bones together.

Little League elbow. Pain in the elbow from throwing too much by a young athlete whose growth plates have not yet closed; can cause permanent damage.

Medial. Inside.

Medial collateral ligament/lateral collateral ligament (MCL/ LCL). The knee ligaments that provide stability for side-to-side movements.

Meniscus. Cartilage plates in the knee between the femur (thigh-bone) and tibia (lower leg bone).

MRI (magnetic resonance imaging). A computer-generated image that uses a magnetic field to show the soft tissues (tendon, ligament, muscle, and cartilage) and their injuries.

Muscular back pain. Pain along the sides of the spine from muscles that are too weak to function properly; often worsens with torso rotation.

Nutritional supplements. A broad category of substances — none of which has ever been tested by the FDA (Food and Drug Administration) — that athletes (and nonathletes) take to improve performance. None of these compounds has been tested in children or teens, and the long-term safety is not known. Products include creatine, androstenedione, HMB, and ma juang.

Overuse injury. Injury from repetitive activity, which causes tissue breakdown. Athletes complain of pain that seems to worsen over time. Most overuse injuries are preventable with good preseason conditioning and proper biomechanics.

Patella. Kneecap.

Patellofemoral knee pain. The most common type of knee pain. Occurs in the front of the knee, underneath the patella.

Physiologic development. Changes in the body's ability to tolerate longer and longer periods of exercise, measured by $VO_{2\,Max}$ (maximum oxygen extraction).

Power lifting. Maximum weight lifting, trying to "max out" for two or three repetitions. Not safe for kids or teens due to potential for growth-plate injury.

Preseason conditioning. Getting in shape for the sports season, starting about six weeks before practice begins. Should address both cardiovascular and muscular conditioning.

Pronation. Rolling in of the arch of the foot; flat-footedness.

Protein. One of the three energy-producing nutrients, available from plants as well as animals. The body uses protein to build and repair muscle. Most adolescents don't get enough protein in their diet.

Psychological development. Changes in the developing psyche of the adolescent toward autonomy and independence that make a person unique and provide a sense of self.

RICE (**R**est, **I**ce, **C**ompression, **E**levation). Treatment of injured ankle or knee during the first twenty-four to forty-eight hours after injury.

Rotator cuff muscles. Four muscles that work in unison inside the shoulder to provide stability during throwing and overhead movements.

Rotator cuff tendinitis. Inflammation of the rotator cuff tendons that frequently occurs in swimmers, tennis players, and baseball players.

Rupture. A complete tear of a ligament.

Sexual development. The maturation of teens that prepares the body to reproduce, manifested in visible changes such as breast development in girls and facial hair and deepening voice in boys; these visible changes are also called secondary sex characteristics.

Shoulder. Joint with greatest range of motion in the body and frequent site of injury for athletes such as tennis players and baseball players. Made up of four joints; glenohumeral joint and acromio-clavicular joint are most commonly injured in sports.

Skeletal development. Changes in the growing skeleton, including muscles and bones, that parallel sexual development.

Spondylolysis. Stress fracture in the spine; often worsens with bending backward.

Sprain. Partial tearing of a ligament.

Strain. Muscle injury; partial tearing of the muscle.

Strength training. Weight lifting using light weights and many repetitions to build strength. Safe for kids and teens, but needs to be supervised by adults.

Stress fracture. Overuse injury of a bone that results when too much stress is placed on it, causing its cortex (outside layer) to crack.

Stress injury. Precursor of a stress fracture. The cortex of the bone is irritated but does not crack. Stress injury is easier to treat than stress fracture.

Subluxation. The slipping of a joint out of the socket then back into place. This is often treated with rehabilitation to increase muscular strength.

Tendinitis. Overuse injury of the tendon, such as Achilles tendinitis.

Vitamins and minerals. Nutrients that provide no energy but that are essential in helping energy-producing nutrients function properly in the body. The body cannot produce vitamins and minerals on its own and needs to ingest them from food sources.

X-ray. Diagnostic test that shows bones but not soft tissue such as tendons, ligaments, muscles, and cartilage.

Notes

Chapter 1. The Benefits of Youth Sports

Why kids play sports. *Care of the Young Athlete*, ed. J. Andy Sullivan, M.D., and Steven J. Anderson, M.D. (Elk Grove, Ill.: American Academy of Orthopaedic Surgeons and American Academy of Pediatrics, 2000), p. 3.

Researchers at Michigan State University: Martha E. Ewing, Vern D. Seefeldt, and Tempie P. Brown, "The Role of Organized Sport in the Education and Health of American Children and Youth," in *The Role of Sports in Youth Development: Report of a Meeting Convened by Carnegie Corporation of New York, March 18, 1996*, ed. Alex Poinsett (New York: Carnegie Corporation, 1996), p. 3. This very readable report cites numerous studies on youth sports, as does Ronald Jeziorski's *The Importance of School Sports in American Education and Socialization* (Lanham, Md.: University Press of America, 1994). Another study of sports that compiles a variety of studies is Andrew W. Miracle, Jr., and C. Roger Rees, *Lessons of the Locker Room: The Myth of School Sports* (Amherst, N.Y.: Prometheus Books, 1994); as might be inferred from its title, the authors are convinced that no good comes from sports.

How rules work. Ronald E. Smith, Ph.D., Frank L. Smoll, Ph.D., and Nathan J. Smith, M.D., *Parents' Complete Guide to Youth Sports* (Costa Mesa, Calif.: HDL Publishing, 1989), p. 27.

The President's Council. The President's Council on Physical Fitness and Sports Report, *Physical Activity and Sport in the Lives of Girls: Physical and Mental Health Dimensions from an Interdisciplinary Approach,* Executive Summary, 1997. Washington, D.C., www.fitness.gov/girlssports.html. "The results are striking: regular physical activity can reduce girls' risk of many of the chronic diseases of adulthood; female athletes do better academically and have lower school dropout rates than their nonathletic counterparts; and regular physical activity can enhance girls' mental health, reducing symptoms of stress and depression and improving self-esteem" (Message from the President's Council on Physical Fitness and Sports). This paper is an overview of research in the field, draws forthright conclusions, and recommends policy and research initiatives.

Women's Sports Foundation. Women's Sports Foundation, Eisenhower Park, East Meadow, New York 11554, www.WomenSportsFoundation.org.

Carol Gilligan. *In a Different Voice: Psychological Theory and Women's Development* (Cambridge, Mass.: Harvard University Press, 1982).

Mike Nerney can be reached at mcnerney@capital.net.

Changing physiology. James McBride Dabbs with Mary Godwin Dabbs, in *Heroes, Rogues, and Lovers* (New York: McGraw-Hill, 2000), documented this phenomenon in an experiment testing Brazilian and Italian soccer fans before and after a World Cup soccer match.

Chapter 3. Put Me In, Coach

Girls are interested in social relationships: See Carol Gilligan, *In a Different Voice.*

Anson Dorrance. *Sports Illustrated,* December 7, 1998.

Chapter 5. The Developing Athlete

Ego identity. "The sense of ego identity . . . is the accrued confidence that the inner sameness and continuity prepared in the past are matched by the sameness and continuity of one's meaning for others, as evidenced in the tangible promise of a 'career.'" Erik H. Erikson, *Childhood and Society*, 2nd ed. (New York: Norton, 1963).

Chapter 6. Nutrition and Nutritional Supplements

Diuretics are unhealthy. R. Hickner, C. Horswill, J. Welker, J. Scott, J. Roemmich, and D. Costill, "Test Development for the Study of Physical Performance in Wrestlers Following Weight Loss," *International Journal of Sports Medicine* 12 (6) (1991): 557–62.

Further Reading

Parenting and Coaching

Smith, Ronald E., Ph.D., Frank L. Smoll, Ph.D., and Nathan J. Smith, M.D. *Parents' Complete Guide to Youth Sports.* Costa Mesa, Calif.: HDL Publishing, 1989.

> An excellent introduction to youth sports, this book offers a very sensible overview of injuries, nutrition, drugs, and college. It gives particular attention to the psychological issues of athletes, both outstanding and average (two of the authors are psychologists).

Sullivan, J. Andy, M.D., and Steven J. Anderson, M.D., eds. *Care of the Young Athlete.* Elk Grove, Ill.: American Academy of Pediatrics and American Academy of Orthopaedic Surgeons, 2000.

> A comprehensive treatment of sports written for doctors, it includes benefits, risks, psychological and physical development, training, injuries, sports and disabilities, cardiac conditions, and more. If parents have a special interest in particular medical conditions or injuries, they can consult this book, although they will have to wade through language such as

"Inversion is a less stable position for the ankle than eversion because the lengths of the medial and lateral malleoli differ."

Thompson, Jim. *Positive Coaching: Building Character and Self-Esteem Through Sports.* Portola Valley, Calif.: Warde Publishers, 1995.

An outstanding book that addresses coaches. And it offers just what the subtitle says: tips on how to build character and self-esteem through sports. Thompson has created a national program based at Stanford University that helps coaches encourage and support kids rather than tear them down, founded on redefining winning (focus on effort and improvement rather than the score) and a method to chart positive versus negative comments. The book is full of good ideas but is very long.

Women's Sports Foundation, Eisenhower Park, East Meadow, New York 11554, 800-227-3988, www.WomensSportsFoundation.org.

This nonprofit organization, founded in 1974 by tennis great Billie Jean King, is dedicated to increasing the participation of girls and women in sports and fitness. It is an invaluable source of information on everything from Title IX issues, to "Images and Words in Women's Sports," to "Health Risks and the Teen Athlete."

Sports

Bissinger, H. G. *Friday Night Lights: A Town, a Team, and a Dream.* New York: DaCapo Press, 1990.

High school football in West Texas, where winning, and going to state, is the most important thing in town. On Friday nights in hardscrabble Odessa, the Permian Panthers draw as many as twenty thousand fans. Bissinger vividly describes the players, the games, the fans, the economy and sociology of Odessa, but most of all, the passion for football.

Geist, Bill. *Little League Confidential: One Coach's Completely Unauthorized Tale of Survival.* New York: Macmillan, 1992.

A droll, loving, observant recounting of small-town Little League, told by coach and master journalist Bill Geist. Anyone with a child playing organized sports will recognize the kids, the parents, the coaches, the situations, the skulduggery Geist describes. This is a cult classic.

Lefkowitz, Bernard. *Our Guys*. New York: Vintage, 1997.

The nightmare version of sports, this is the story of the Glen Ridge, New Jersey, high school football players who raped a mentally retarded girl in 1989. Here the law of the jungle prevails (the strong brutalize and humiliate the weak) and adult intervention is virtually nonexistent. The author doesn't have a good word to say about the town or the people who live there.

McGinniss, Joe. *The Miracle of Castel di Sangro*. Boston: Little, Brown, 1999.

One man's obsession with minor-league Italian soccer. This gripping book describes the culture of small-town, backwater Italy and the fortunes of a team trying to make it to the next level. Soccer lovers have difficulty pulling themselves away from this book.

College

Wheeler, Dion. *A Parent's and Student-Athlete's Guide to Athletic Scholarships*. Lincolnwood, Ill.: Contemporary Books, 2000.

This book offers a lot of useful information about sports and college, including a glossary and a list of colleges with each one's mailing address, sports programs by gender, affiliation, and phone number of the athletic director.

Shulman, James E., and William G. Bowen. *The Game of Life: College Sports and Educational Values*. Princeton: Princeton University Press, 2001.

For readers interested in the complexities of collegiate athletics and academic policy. The Mellon Foundation has constructed a detailed database of student records from twenty-eight selective colleges and universities. In *The Shape of the River* (Princeton University Press, 1998), the precursor to *The Game of Life*, William Bowen (former president of Princeton) and Derek Bok (former president of Harvard) research the database and promote the role of affirmative action. They find that African Americans get a boost with admissions at these schools. They earn below-average grades and less money than their white classmates, but they become leaders in the community (defined as participation in civic organizations). The increased diversity in the student body and "special obligation to educate larger numbers of minority students who could then be expected to play leadership roles in the mainstream of American life . . . relate directly to the educational mission of these institutions" (*Game of Life*, p. 85).

In *The Game of Life*, Bowen and Shulman research the same database and denigrate the role of intercollegiate athletics. They find that athletes get a boost with admissions, earn below-average grades, are more conservative than students-at-large (evidently a form of diversity to be discouraged), earn more than fellow students-at-large, but do not become leaders (defined in this case as being a CEO, entering public service, or participating in civic leadership), although former athletes do have higher participation rates as leaders of youth groups and as trustees and advocates for their alma maters than students-at-large do. The authors believe that given these outcomes, athletes consume too many "institutional resources—money, admissions slots, and administration time" (p. 27). Most of their concerns are in the "high profile" sports of football and basketball. These concerns could be alleviated by decreasing the number of roster spots on a school's football team, since football, by itself, accounts for 26 to 45 percent of expenditures on athletics at Division I-A schools. This solution is unfeasible for large public universities dependent on the enthusiasm of state legislators and their constituents but may well be possible for smaller private institutions working collaboratively.

Index